D0486518

Unveiling Depression in Women

Unveiling
Depression
in Women

**A Practical Guide to Understanding
and Overcoming Depression**

Archibald Hart, Ph.D.
Catherine Hart Weber, Ph.D.

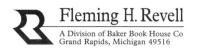

Fleming H. Revell
A Division of Baker Book House Co
Grand Rapids, Michigan 49516

© 2002 by Archibald Hart, Ph.D., and Catherine Hart Weber, Ph.D.

Published by Fleming H. Revell
a division of Baker Book House Company
P.O. Box 6287, Grand Rapids, MI 49516-6287

Third printing, October 2003

Printed in the United States of America

All rights reserved. No part of this publication may be reproduced, stored in a retrieval system, or transmitted in any form or by any means—for example, electronic, photocopy, recording—without the prior written permission of the publisher. The only exception is brief quotations in printed reviews.

Library of Congress Cataloging-in-Publication Data
Hart, Archibald D.
    Unveiling depression in women : a practical guide to understanding and overcoming depression / Archibald Hart, Catherine Hart Weber.
        p.   cm.
    Includes bibliographical references.
    ISBN 0-8007-5749-1(pbk.)
    1. Depression in women. 2. Depression in women—Religious aspects—Christianity. I. Weber, Catherine Hart, 1975-II. Title.
RC537 .H3545 2002
616.85′27′0082—dc21   2001059617

Unless otherwise marked, Scripture is taken from the HOLY BIBLE, NEW INTERNATIONAL VERSION®. Copyright © 1973, 1978, 1984, by International Bible Society. Used by permission of Zondervan Publishing House. All rights reserved.

Scripture marked NASB is from the NEW AMERICAN STANDARD BIBLE®. Copyright © The Lockman Foundation 1960, 1962, 1963, 1968, 1971, 1972, 1973, 1975, 1977, 1995. Used by permission.

For current information about all releases from Baker Book House, visit our web site:
                    http://www.bakerbooks.com

This book is lovingly dedicated
to all the young girls and women in our families:
Kathleen, Catherine, Sharon, Sylvia,
Nicole, Ashley, and Caitlan

Contents

Introduction

Chances are, you've been touched by depression in some way. It's an epidemic, after all, especially among women and children. In fact, every fourth woman around you has the potential for becoming seriously depressed; if you're that woman, you only have a one in three chance of getting the help you really need. Too many women will suffer alone unnecessarily, hoping somehow they'll snap out of it.

Whether you're that woman with firsthand experience of depression or simply close to someone who fights it, there's no need to feel alone or helpless.

This book can help you.

It's an updated, comprehensive, practical resource and guide that shows, explains, and gives tools for overcoming and building resistance to mild to moderate depression. Along with the latest medical, psychological, and practical information, it offers a biblical approach and our prayer that through a proper understanding of God's divine plan for your health and wholeness, you'll discover complete healing.

Keep in mind that if you or someone you know is experiencing severe clinical depression or has been depressed for some time, it's important to get competent, qualified professional help to determine the cause and severity. Counseling, along with possible antidepressant medication, social support, and a wellness lifestyle, will be essential for a full recovery and for preventing a relapse.

To help you each step of the way, this book aims to keep things simple and give you just the information you need. In fact, if you're too daunted right now to even delve into the entire book from front to back, start just with this summary. You'll find the chapters supporting these summary points are full of more detailed and useful help.

1. *Depression is treatable!* See chapter 1. Get help as soon as you can. The longer you wait, the harder it gets.
2. *You need not be alone—talk to someone you trust.* Encouragement, support, and help can be found when you confide any thoughts about how you're feeling.
3. *You can know the severity of your depression and determine its type.* Take the depression quiz in chapter 2; if your depression is moderate to severe, seek professional help immediately.
4. *You can understand the underlying cause(s) of your depression and what it may be signaling to you.* A thorough medical and psychological evaluation will help determine risk factors, and chapters 3 to 6 address these.
5. *You can know the most effective treatment options for you,* whether it's counseling and psychotherapy; antidepressant medication therapy for moderate to severe and long-term depression; or other natural complementary treatment options and remedies, including wellness lifestyle choices for preventing future depressions. See chapters 7 to 10.
6. *You can get treatment—and quickly.* Your doctor or a friend can help if you've experienced depression symptoms for more than two weeks, if your depression is affecting your life in negative ways, or if you are having thoughts or feelings of hurting yourself. Call a suicide hot line or have someone take you to an emergency room if you are not able to go yourself. Always remember: Your problem might be physical and easily treated.

7. *A professional counselor can help you on an ongoing basis* by helping you discover and heal some deep-seated emotional hurt, or more positively aligning your beliefs, thoughts, and behaviors.

8. *You can receive a complete medical examination that rules out other possible physical or medical conditions that could be causing your depression.* Your doctor can give you the appropriate referral for treatment of any underlying physical problem.

9. *A positive support system is just a phone call away.* Family, friends, your church community, and others close to you can take you to appointments or help you with the necessities of daily living. Take advantage of this as it will help you find connections during this painful time.

10. *You can take small steps every day that move you toward strategies for recovery.* Chapter 10 guides you through practical resources for overcoming depression and for wellness living. We also equip you for the roadblocks to your recovery.

11. *You can learn how to live with a woman who is depressed.* Tools in chapter 11 show you how to be helpful, as well as how to care for yourself.

Finally, know that this guide aims to help you become knowledgeable enough to be your own health advocate. We'll guide you through getting the professional help you need, as well as taking care of yourself and making healthy lifestyle choices. And the result is something you can take heart in: With each new thing you learn, test, and try, you will be on the road to recovery and building your resistance to future depressions.

PART 1 | Understanding Depression in Women

1

What Every Woman Should Know

Why are you downcast, O my soul, my inner self?
Why are you so disturbed and disquieted within me?
I choose to put my hope in you, God, to wait expectantly
    for you, and I will still praise You, my help, my Savior
    and my God.
O my God, my life is downcast within me, and it is more
    than I can bear; therefore I will earnestly remember you!

                                    Prayer inspired by Psalm 42:5–6

Nena is the envy of many. A charming, warm, and happy
forty-two-year-old, she completed college with top hon-
ors and took up teaching as a career. She can sew, crochet,
cook, bake, paint in watercolors, and enjoy a good laugh.
She is a very good mother, wife, neighbor, and Christian,
and is highly sought after to be on every church commit-
tee imaginable. Outwardly, there is nothing wrong with
her life. She is adored by a doting husband and lovingly
respected by her two teenage children, a boy and a girl.

But the outside doesn't always match the inside. One
day while getting out of bed, Nena felt something wasn't
"right." At first, she considered it a mild case of the flu, but
things got worse. It wasn't the flu at all.

A profound state of fatigue had overtaken her, and it continued to the point that mornings brought an endless fight to get out of bed. Nena had once been an early riser, often going for a jog with her husband before getting the kids ready and off to school. But now that seemed impossibly far away. She would just lie there, feeling that her arms and legs couldn't respond to her wishes.

Nena also noticed that she was somewhat irritable and would burst into tears at the slightest provocation. Throughout the day, she would find herself overcome with intense sadness she couldn't explain. There was no reason for it. Her life was so perfect. She tried not to alarm her husband and kept much of what she was feeling to herself. At times, though, he would ask her if everything was okay, and she would reassure him that it was, saying something like, "I'm just feeling a little under the weather. Must be a touch of the flu."

Nena tried to force herself to do things. She continued teaching, though it was becoming more difficult each day. She'd collapse on her bed the moment she arrived home and increasingly did not have meals prepared on time. She withdrew from the family. Finally, her husband sat her down and expressed concern about the changes he had seen taking place over the last few months. Nena conceded something was wrong.

It was the family doctor who diagnosed Nena's depression. He'd known her for a long time and immediately noticed the change. It was something in her eyes.

By clinical standards, Nena's depression was mild. Despite becoming somewhat incapacitated by it, she was able to put on a brave face to the outside world. None of her friends realized she was depressed, and only those as close as her family had wondered if something was wrong.

Her treatment was quite straightforward. A medical evaluation showed that she was in perimenopause, a time when estrogen levels begin to decline, and a family history revealed that her mother had suffered from a severe menopausal depression which had never been treated. Her doctor referred her to a psychologist for counseling, and after consulting with her gynecologist, placed her on an antidepressant medication. The result? Nena is once again a vitally alive, vivacious, and charming person.

For Nena, depression stemmed from reproductive problems. Whatever the cause of the depression, however, the story is repeated again and again, in every neighborhood of every city.

Big-Time Blues

Life is full of emotional ups and downs. At times everyone experiences the "blues," and nearly every woman, at some time in her life, will experience a mild to serious form of depression that might even be incapacitating. Surprised? There's a wide variety of depression out there, ranging from normal experiences that get better by themselves to clinical depressions like Nena's, which actually need treatment. Unfortunately, the clinical type can be quite disruptive, and it's becoming increasingly more common in women today. It's absolutely essential, then, that women educate themselves about the possible risks.

A good place to start is with an understanding of "normal" depression, and the reasons it's so common. The pace of life, chronic stress, relationship conflicts, hurts, rejections, and the ups and downs of the immune system all wreak havoc with our moods. But these are the "normal" consequences of being human. People are designed to experience sadness and grief whenever encountering a loss of any sort. Furthermore, women's bodies are constantly adjusting to hormonal fluctuations, especially at times of childbirth and illness. Loved ones get sick or die, and our dreams don't always pan out. The result is that feelings of disappointment, devastation, and even despair are par for the course of life. But sometimes, maybe even often, normal depressions erupt into more serious and debilitating episodes. The good news is, with God's help, there is no reason why your depression can't become a healing experience, allowing you to take great steps toward maturity in your personal and spiritual life.

A Little Stress Never Hurt, Did It?

Every mother knows about stress. Mothers have to deal with a constant flow of pressures and the "chronic strain of the mundane," everyday home management, baby nurturing, and toddler parenting, not to mention the care of teenagers and husbands. On top of this, many women also have to work outside of the home. Despite the benefits, that work undoubtedly adds further strain to an already overstrained body. Balancing the demands of family, work, and caring for yourself can be overwhelming. Some women who are single parents have to face these challenges alone, and they deserve real admiration.

These demands are all a part of modern life, and they don't necessarily lead to clinical depression. That doesn't mean we should underestimate their effects. The cumulative outcome of trying to survive while keeping up with the rest of the human race, with no opportunity for respite, can lead to a devastating depression.

"Kindling" for the Fire

Okay, so you're mildly depressed. But how long has it been going on? When even a mild depression is allowed to continue for many months or years, the symptoms may slowly increase in severity through a phenomenon called "kindling." As you probably know, kindling is what makes it easier to light fires, and this is just what prolonged "little" depressions can do. When not acknowledged or effectively treated, these little depressions can turn into a seemingly endless dark cloud that starts to interfere with your basic life functioning.

Understanding Depression

Clinical depressions are also called mood or affective disorders. There are no biological tests for depression, so the diagnosis is usually a matter of recognizing its various forms by the cluster of symptoms associated with each. The most recognizable symptom is an abnormal change in mood, which is where the label "mood disorder" comes from.

While depression may be limited to mood changes, it is considered a whole-person disorder since the body, mind, emotions, relationships, and spirituality are all affected.

The *mind* is affected because depression lowers attention span, tolerance for frustration, and memory. *Behavior* is affected by lowered motivation, loss of ability to experience pleasure, and fatigue. The *body* is affected by headaches, stomach aches, and muscle tension. *Relationships* are affected by a tendency to withdraw and become isolated with loneliness. Lowered impulse control can lead to suicide or homicide. Depression can also create sleep disturbances, changes in appetite and weight, and lowered sex drive.

Depression can appear suddenly and for no apparent reason, or it may be triggered by a variety of causes such as illness, hormonal fluctuations, or the season of the year. Ongoing struggles, such as trying to overcome abuse, can aggravate any depression. Some have only one episode in a lifetime; others have recurring episodes.

Overall, depression is considered "clinical" when symptoms are severe and include difficulty getting through a daily routine, sleeping too much or too little, disturbance of concentration, excessive negative or pessimistic thoughts, severe guilt, and an inability to connect with or be around others. Secondary symptoms include diverse aches and pains, headaches, or other uncomfortable physical symptoms. Depression can make you feel overwhelmed, anxious, worthless, and hopeless, and you might even have thoughts about ending your life.

Unfortunately, as severe as these symptoms sound, many women don't realize they're depressed. They may simply visit their doctor complaining of uncomfortable physical symptoms, or may see a psychotherapist because of family relationship conflicts or other lifestyle problems. As such, many of these depressions are masked by other complaints.

If left untreated, depression can become serious. It can rob people from many hours of effective functioning—and sometimes rob them of life itself. At any given time, it is estimated that up to 20 percent of the population have disturbed daily functioning due to clinical depression. If you find yourself in this category and have experienced any of these symptoms for longer than two weeks, seek professional help. We'll look at what kinds of help are available in coming chapters.

Why Do I Feel This Way?

There are many theories about what causes depression, and all together, they can be rather confusing. Individually, however, each theory has contributed something to our understanding.

For example, some theorists believe that depression is anger turned inward. The "learned helplessness" model, on the other hand, attributes depression to habitual patterns of pessimism and hopelessness. And as for the "medical model," it explains depression as the result of biochemical imbalances in the brain, comparing it to other medical illnesses like diabetes, chronic asthma, or even heart disease. In other words, you can't just "snap out of it" or resolve your illness by being strong. Depression, like any other illness, needs to be treated.

There are other theories, as well. Some believe that depression is a response to the losses in life, such as a grief experienced in bereavement, and is actually an attempt to avoid pain. And then there's the cognitive theory, which attributes depression to distorted thinking processes. Still others believe that depression can be like a "darkness" that comes out of nowhere for no apparent reason, engulfing you when you least expect it.

As you can see, there's no simple explanation for depression. A given case could be associated with, triggered by, or caused by any of these factors. It may even be a combination of several.

What we do know, following many years of scientific research, is that depression is a complex, interrelated disorder, and its symptoms include a wide variety of discomforts.

Whether depression is classified as an illness, disease, disorder, or syndrome, the underlying causes are complexly interrelated. They have origins in your body, genes, temperament, pattern of thinking, way of handling emotions, family history, relationships, and past and current experience. As such, it's truly a whole-body, whole-person disorder, and for treatment to be effective, it must also be comprehensive. Medication can be helpful to some women, but it is not always a sufficient treatment for depression. Alone, it should never be thought of as a "cure."

For your recovery to be complete, it will be important for you to understand the underlying cause(s) of your depression. It will also be important for you to actively participate in a comprehensive treatment plan, which may include antidepressant medications, counseling, and attention to your own self care and a healthy lifestyle.

An Epidemic on the Rise

According to current research, more and more women and children are getting depressed. They're also becoming more severely depressed, and they're starting at an earlier age than ever before. In each successive generation, depression is likely to begin at younger and younger ages, and over the course of a lifetime, the risk of depression keeps increasing.[1]

For the baby boomer generation, or those born after 1940, the number of people that were depressed by the age of 25 is in the tens of millions. Studies show that people born in the second half of the century are 10 times more likely to suffer from depression than people born in the first half. Adolescents are the fastest growing age group affected, but those between 25 and 45 are the largest group already suffering depression.[2]

To explain this increase, we will explore the explanations in chapter 3. But to begin with, lets take a closer look at our contemporary culture and lifestyle. Richard Swenson suggests that "the answer lies in the fact that we have been ambushed by a load of psychic trauma unparalleled in human history. . . . Never before have people faced the particular constellation of factors which today are plotting together for our misery."[3]

Modern life is bombarded with anxiety, stress and overload, and this wages war on our emotions. Stress and anxiety seem to have a high association with depression. Life goes along at top speed, and it seems almost impossible to adapt and keep up. In addition, families are fractured and in disarray, and our lives are more mobile, which makes community and social support sparse. Children suffer from the emotional trauma of abuse, neglect, and shifting family values and structures as a result of divorce. Our teens are faced with more negative media and cultural influence, leading to a rise in substance abuse, teenage pregnancy, pornography or sexual addiction, and crime. And let's not forget that more people are experiencing financial problems, with more debt than ever before.

Just the Facts, Ma'am

So just how big is the problem of depression among women? In the United States alone, millions of women currently have diagnosed clinical depression. In addition:

- Only one out of every three women who experience clinical depression will seek care.
- Married women have higher rates of depression than unmarried women.
- Girls entering puberty are twice as prone to depression as boys.
- Elderly women experience depression more often than elderly men.
- Depression is the leading cause of disability in women.
- Research shows a strong relationship between eating disorders and depression.
- Depression usually occurs along with chronic stress and anxiety.
- Depression tends to recur for many women.

- Almost 15 percent of all those suffering from severe depression will commit suicide.

Women Get Depressed More Than Men

As you can see, if you're now—or ever have been—depressed, or if you know of a woman who is, you're in good company. At least one study stated that 21.3 percent of American women had experienced at least one major depressive episode during their lifetime.

It is now widely accepted that women are two to three times more likely than men to report suffering from depression, and this applies all over the world. Depression has been called the most significant health risk for women, with younger women of childbearing and childrearing age being the greatest targets.[4]

Studies done in Canada, Puerto Rico, Paris, and West Germany have all concluded that about twice as many women have had serious depression episodes than men. The only exception seems to be within the Amish and Jewish populations. In these communities, alcoholism is less frequent than in the population at large, but rates of depression are the same for men and women. This may have to do with the expectation that men feel and express their emotions more openly, therefore lowering their chances for masked and "acting out" depressive behaviors. Another explanation could be that, due to the strong social support and extended families that these communities provide, the vulnerability to social isolation is much reduced, greatly lowering the rate of depression for their women. It is also speculated that the role of women in the home and family is greatly valued and appreciated, and that this lowers the ongoing frustration and social pressures that puts other women at risk for depression—a lesson that our greater culture could heed. Many other explanations continue to be explored.

There Is a Light at the End of the Tunnel

Regardless of the cause of a specific depression, research and clinical evidence show that depression is treatable. Unfortunately, too many depressed women suffer needlessly because they don't realize they can be helped.

Much misunderstanding and stigma have been attached to depression, especially when it comes to women. Depressed women have been made to feel ashamed that they were weak, and many have become so frustrated with the helping professions that they avoid treatment altogether. The church hasn't exactly helped, either, in some cases adding guilt or not being supportive of counseling or antidepressant medication. Many have been made to feel that they have somehow failed God. *Aren't strong enough to follow this will,*

As if all this wasn't enough, depression is often misdiagnosed. Many of its symptoms, such as fatigue, sleep disturbances, and weight change, mimic those of other diseases. This can make the diagnosis of depression difficult, and if it's not diagnosed correctly, women go away frustrated, still wondering what's wrong.

This means that many women with depression do not know they are depressed. They might end up being treated for problems like insomnia, headaches, pain problems, anxiety, fatigue, or stress-related symptoms. Often they are given useless medications or end up self-medicating with alcohol, drugs, sex, and relationships. The Agency for Health Care Policy and Research reports that only one-third to one-half of women with major depressive disorder are properly diagnosed by medical practitioners. Other women never even seek help or treatment, hoping they'll just get over it, suffering through the unnecessary difficulty and pain of severe symptoms.

How Does God Fit?

God has designed us with the capacity for experiencing depression. Just as pain is important for the survival of the body because it alerts us to harm and disease, depression alerts us to something out of order in the physical, emotional, or mental realm. It has been said that "depression is a cry in the soul that something is missing."

While severe depression is totally mysterious for the one experiencing it—and in many respects caused by some biological abnormality—the lesser depressions can be purposeful. Consider, for example, reactive depression, which is a response to loss. We are designed by God to respond to loss with grief. It's our way of saying good-bye to that which has been taken from us.

Making the Pain Redemptive

So, while depression can be very painful at times, it does serve a purpose. Many therapists are now drawing attention to the fact that depression is adaptive, meaning that some good can come out of it.

Simply getting rid of the symptom of anxiety or any other uncomfortable and painful symptoms won't bring long-term relief, recovery, growth, and wellness. Life is difficult enough as it is. A redemptive perspective will help you learn how to handle these difficult circumstances with grace and fruitfulness so that they do not become destructive to your life or relationships. You can learn and change in positive ways during these times. For one thing, depression can teach you empathy and concern for others. As you move through the pain, you can experience enrich-ment, growth, maturity, and depth of character. The great-est gain could be enriching intimacy in your relationship with God and the people around you.

2

Recognizing Depression

I wait, expect, look for, and hope in you, Lord, to renew
  my strength and power;
so I can be up close to you, God, like eagles are up close to
  the sun;
so I can run and not be weary and walk and not faint and
  become tired.

Prayer inspired by Isaiah 40:31

You might say mild depression is the common cold of our
emotions. With all the challenges that life can bring, including sadness, pain, loss, stress, uncertainty, rejection,
disappointments, physical illness, change, and distorted
pessimistic feelings, it's no wonder that 25 percent of us
are feeling it at any given moment.

This mild, sometimes called "normal," depression may
rob us of a zest for life, but it's not a serious condition.
In fact, many experts are convinced mild depression is
"adaptive," and that it actually makes us stronger. It has
the same effect on us that wind has on trees. If trees are
sheltered from strong winds when growing, they put
down shallow roots that make them vulnerable to being
blown over by stronger winds at a later time. In other

words, that mild depression can strengthen our coping skills, making us more resilient for whatever's coming next.

Sometimes, however, that resiliency weakens. The depression may last longer or get deeper, and that's when normal depression needs the sort of help we are offering here. As a general rule, when a period of pronounced sadness persists for more than two weeks, you may actually have a clinical depression, and this is when you should consider getting help.

The Big Picture

Since for every depressed person there are at least three others whose lives have been significantly affected, and since it has been said that, by the year 2020, depression will be the greatest disability worldwide, what can be done? Start by learning what type of depression you're dealing with, since not all depressions are the same, and they certainly don't present all the same symptoms.

Different Depression, Different Causes

It's important to note that not all mental health professionals agree about the categories of depression. While depression goes back to the earliest of times—for example, there are many classic descriptions of depression in Scripture—it was only recently that we discovered different depressions can have different causes. Just one hundred years ago, the biological causes were unknown. In fact, all depression was attributed to psychological causes. So let us make a clear statement here: While some depressions have psychological, environmental, or even spiritual causes, other depressions have biological origins. They are physical illnesses. Yes, there are stress factors, but these tend to aggravate rather than cause depression. We want to emphasize this because so many women feel guilty for being depressed, as if they are somehow to blame for it.

The main publication used by mental health specialists to describe and diagnose mood disorders, known as the *Diagnostic and Statistical Manual of Mental Disorders (DSM-IV)*, describes depression according to the severity of symptoms, not by etiology. In other words, it does not try to describe the causes of depression, whether they are related to hormones, genetics, or situations. It is left to the treating professional to figure out specific causes, which is why it is important to seek out professional help, not just diagnose yourself.

Using three simple categories, *DSM-IV* classifies depression as *unipolar,* lasting for more than two weeks; *bipolar,* if it includes mania; or *dysthymia,* which is long term and chronic. The mental health specialist then determines cause and severity. If the symptoms are severe, the depression is considered "major affective disorder."

We'd like to take a slightly different approach. Looking more at the cause of a depression than its severity, we can place it in one of two categories: biologically based or psychologically/socially based. Biologically based depressions, including those caused by genetics, hormones, or disease, are essentially the result of changes in brain chemistry. In general, they respond well to medications. Psychologically or socially based depressions, on the other hand, relate to emotional, mental, spiritual, or relational issues. Since there's nothing wrong with brain chemistry in these depressions, antidepressants play a minimal role in treating these. Psychotherapy is the preferred modality.

Biologically based depressions are sometimes called "endogenous depressions," meaning that they originate "from within" your body. Psychologically/socially based depressions are called "exogenous" or "reactive" depressions, because they originate "from without." They are a response to life's circumstances such as bereavement, loss, disappointment, and stress.

No matter what the type of depression, however, once it sets in, it impacts all areas of life. Let's look at Jeanne's case to illustrate. Jeanne is a thirty-five-year-old graphic artist with two small girls. As a single mother, she has her hands full. She also suffers from a long-standing deficient thyroid gland, a common biological cause of depression in women. Jeanne has pretty consistently resisted taking her thyroid supplement, often allowing the prescription to run out. So, while she is depressed primarily because of her thyroid condition, it doesn't stop there. Her depression also impacts her effectiveness at work. At times she is quite irritable, and this causes increased relational stress for her. Her job problems impact her job security, so much so that she has become extremely insecure in her work. Of course, if she loses her job, she will be in serious financial trouble. And that increased anxiety has begun to affect the quality of her work. She does not feel as creative as before, and her creativity is in rapid decline. Domino Effect

Jeanne's case is a clear example of emotional "chaining," in which a sequence of losses is created, one loss giving rise to another, and each loss causing more depression that is added to the primary depression. Jeanne became even more disillusioned, hopeless, and depressed, not from the original biological factor, but from all the other psychological/social factors that followed. Finally, she sought help and was able to get her life back on track again. But her story demonstrates that even a small, physically caused depression that is untreated can lead to serious social and vocational consequences.

Types of Depression

Here's a breakdown of the more common types of depression, so you'll better understand what we're talking about:

- *Unipolar depression:* This is also known as clinical or major depression. It's the most common form of depression, affecting over fifteen million Americans. "Unipolar" means there is no mania, just depressed mood, plus loss of ability to experience pleasure (anhedonia) and feelings of worthlessness, etc., for at least two weeks. In general, this type of depression responds well to medication.

- *Dysthymia:* The same symptoms are present, but are milder, lasting for at least two years and without a break for more than two months. Women with dysthymia can also experience major depressive episodes, which are sometimes called a "double depression." The problem can be treated in the same manner as unipolar.

- *Bipolar depression:* Also known as manic depression. This disorder is not as common as other forms of depression, but still affects about two million Americans. It alternates between severe depression and mania, which is euphoria or irritable excitement, and responds well to medication.

- *Atypical depression:* This involves chronic depression and other symptoms such as excessive fatigue, oversleeping, and overeating. This type of depression is more difficult to treat and may require a combination of medications, which is called "polypharmacy."

- *Seasonal depression:* Women are more susceptible to seasonal affective disorder (SAD) than men, and the episodes can occur throughout a woman's lifetime.

There can be an association between the onset of a major depressive episode and a particular time of the year, usually fall or winter, when there is insufficient sunlight. This is caused by an excess of melatonin, a sleep hormone that is released in the brain with darkness. The depression usually goes into full remission during a particular time of the year, such as spring. It is treated in "light rooms" or "sun rooms," where you can sit under bright lights similar to sunlight for a few hours a day.

Psychotic depression: This is the severest of the depressions because it is accompanied by delusions or hallucinations. It requires immediate psychiatric care. About 15 percent of people with unipolar or bipolar depression are affected.

Hormonal depressions: These include premenstrual dysphoric disorder (PMDD); premenstrual syndrome (PMS); postpartum onset; and perimenopausal depression. These depressions correlate with a drop in estrogen level and often require medical treatment and hormonal replacement therapy in addition to antidepressant medication. In general, about 10 percent of new mothers experience depression.

Post traumatic stress disorder (PTSD): This occurs after exposure to trauma or violence, and symptoms are similar to those for depression. They may also include nightmares, flashbacks of terrifying past events, increased aggression, feelings of uncontrollable anger, emotional numbing, and avoidance of the outside world, especially anything reminiscent of past trauma.

"Masked" depression: While this type is not formally recognized in the diagnostic manual, it is widely acknowledged as very common. It is possible for both men and women to suffer from serious depression and for friends and loved ones not to realize it. The sufferer hides or "masks" it behind some other problem or activity. Instead of complaining of depression, then, they complain about physical problems like indigestion, heartburn, muscle or joint pains, or chronic headaches. Men tend to act out by being more involved with work or outside activities or by becoming angry. Such depressions can go unrecognized, by both the sufferer and loved ones, for a long time.

When considering the different types of depression, remember that a depressed mood follows a continuum, so the feelings associated with it can range from mild to severe. Generally, the more severe a depression, the more likely it is to be endogenous and responsive to antidepressant medications.

Identifying the Symptoms

As with many other conditions, the earlier you catch depression, the easier it is to treat. The following list of symptoms will alert you to the warning signs, and the more of these symptoms you experience, the more severe your depression. We've clustered them according to thoughts, mood, behavior, physical functioning, spiritual factors, and social behavior. Check those which apply to you.

Mood/Emotions
__Depressed mood—feelings of helplessness, worthlessness, sadness, irritability, and pessimism for most of the day

__Excessive crying or an inability to cry or express emotion

__Feelings of worthlessness, hopelessness, inappropriate guilt, or blaming yourself for your problems

__Loss of interest in previously pleasurable activities; inability to enjoy usual hobbies or activities, including sex

__Unresolved grief issues

Changes in mood like those listed above should be the "red flag" that alerts you to depression.

Thoughts

__Inability to concentrate, remember things, make decisions, or think clearly, even on routine tasks

__Obsessing over negative experiences or thoughts

__Low self-esteem

__Recurrent thoughts of suicide or death; you may have already made a will and begun thinking about your funeral

__Feeling pessimistic about your life

__Attitude of, "What difference does it make?"

Physical functioning

__Appetite disturbance, eating far less or far more than usual

__Sleep disturbances—inability to sleep, tossing and turning, not being able to get back to sleep, sleeping too much, or irregular sleep patterns

__Constant fatigue or loss of energy

__Slow, soft speech

__Chronic aches and pains that don't respond to treatment

__Anxiety or panic attacks

__Unexplained headaches, backaches, abdominal pain, constipation, or general aches and pains

Spiritual factors

__Feeling that God is very distant

__Being angry and disappointed in God

__Having no hope for your future

__Feeling abandoned and forsaken by God

__Feeling a heaviness in your spirit

__Feeling like a cloud of darkness is over you

Behavior factors

__Observable restlessness, irritability, or decreased activity

__Substance abuse such as alcohol or drugs

__Suicide attempts

__Decreased performance at work or school

__Social withdrawal—refusal to go out, to see friends, and avoidance of old friends

__Avoidance of situations that could cause responsibility or failure

__Dislike of crowds

__Difficulty getting along with others

As you can see, the list of possible symptoms covers a broad range of human experience. We've provided a depression quiz here so you can dig a little deeper. There are many standardized tests available. This one is called CES-D from the Center for Epidemiological Studies-Depression. It is widely used and was developed by Lenore Radloff at the Center for Epidemiological Studies of the National Institute of Mental Health.

Depression Quiz

To take the quiz, add a point value to each question, according to how you have felt during the past week.

    0   Rarely or none of the time (less than one day)
    1   Some of the time (one or two days)
    2   Occasionally or a moderate amount of the time (three or four days)
    3   Most or all of the time (five to seven days)

1. I was bothered by things that usually don't bother me.
2. I did not feel like eating; my appetite was poor.
3. I felt that I could not shake off the blues even with help from my family and friends.
4. I felt that I was not as good as other people.
5. I had trouble keeping my mind on what I was doing.
6. I felt depressed.
7. I felt that everything I did was an effort.
8. I felt hopeless about the future.
9. I thought my life had been a failure.
10. I felt fearful.
11. My sleep was restless.
12. I was unhappy.
13. I talked less than usual.
14. I felt lonely.
15. People were unfriendly.
16. I did not enjoy life.
17. I had crying spells.
18. I felt sad.
19. I felt that people disliked me.
20. I could not get "going."

To score the test, simply add up the numbers you attributed to each item. The higher the score, the more likely you are depressed.

    0–9:   You are probably not depressed.
    10–15: You may be mildly depressed.
    16–24: You are in the moderately depressed range. Consider getting a professional consultation.
    Over 24: You are probably severely depressed. Seek professional consultation right away.

When taking this quiz, remember that, although it's an accurate tool for determining the symptoms of depression, it's not a definitive diagnosis. Nor does it determine the cause of your depression. It is an example of a standard self-test used to screen for possible depression. Unfortunately, you could have a low score and still be depressed, or a high score and not be clinically depressed. A more accurate diagnosis of depression depends on other factors, such as how long your symptoms have lasted. If your score is in the moderate to severely depressed range, consider getting an accurate professional diagnosis. If you are interested in taking another test, a confidential screening test for clinical depression is available on-line through The National Mental Health Association. Go to www.nmha.org.

In general, an accurate diagnosis of depression requires the following:

- A complete physical examination to rule out the possibility of a physical disorder and the primary cause of depression.
- A complete evaluation by a licensed mental health professional such as a psychologist, psychotherapist, or psychiatrist, who is fully trained in mental health diagnosis and who has sufficient knowledge of medicine to recognize when the symptoms of a mental disorder are due to physical causes and if antidepressant medication is necessary.

Formal Symptoms and Beyond

Sometimes the depression self-screening test can be too general, since it focuses mainly on external symptoms. It can ignore the deeper feelings associated with depression— and it can also ignore the differences between men and women. Atypical symptoms of depression that are more prevalent in women, for example, may include over-sleeping, such as ten to twelve hours a night plus staying in bed longer; increased appetite leading to weight gain; increase in anxiety symptoms; difficulty in making decisions; increased feelings of guilt, especially about things that didn't get accomplished; extreme sensitivity to rejection; and increased self-consciousness.

There can be other symptoms that aren't as easy to describe. Here's what those women used to describe depression:[1]

- Things just seem "off" or "wrong" in your life.
- You don't feel hopeful or happy about anything in your life.
- You feel like you're moving (thinking) in slow motion.
- Getting up in the morning requires a lot of effort.
- Carrying on a normal conversation is a struggle; you can't seem to express yourself.
- Smiling feels stiff and awkward; it's like your smiling muscles are frozen.
- You're forgetful, and it's very difficult to concentrate on anything.
- You have a feeling of impending doom; you think something bad is going to happen, although you may not be sure what.
- In your perception of the world around you, it's always cloudy; even on sunny days, it seems cloudy and gray.
- You feel as though you're drowning or suffocating.
- You're agitated, jumpy, anxious, and worried much of the time.

And how does all this affect your life?

- Your home is a mess—laundry and dishes are piled up, mail is unopened, etc.
- You've been making excuses to friends why you can't get together with them, or you're telling them you're "just too tired."
- You've really let yourself go—you're wearing clothes that make you look dumpy, you've stopped exercising, and you're not shaving unless absolutely necessary.
- You're putting off things that need to be done, such as your car registration, taking a book back to the library, or buying a birthday present for someone.
- You can't remember the last time you laughed a real laugh.
- You've been to the doctor a lot recently, for things like headaches, stomachaches, and fatigue, but the doctor can't find anything wrong. Either that, or you're convinced you have a life-threatening disease.
- You wake up in the middle of the night and can't go back to sleep; during the day you sleep a lot to escape from your life.
- It takes you a whole weekend to do chores that used to only occupy a morning.
- You have no ability to imagine or conceive of your life even a few days ahead and have no plans and no hopes; you can't even be sure you'll still be here.
- You wear the same clothes a few days in a row, since choosing new ones is too much effort.
- You lose track of things and can't always remember what day it is.
- You've pretty much stopped eating or caring what you eat and whether it tastes good.
- On the flip side, you may be eating all the time because you're bored and hope that food will somehow satisfy the vacant feeling you have.
- You've lost interest in sex or even physical affection; hugging someone doesn't feel any different from leaning against a wall.
- You're avoiding talking to anyone to whom you have an obligation, such as your boss or friends.
- You hope you don't run into anyone you know while you're out; not only is maintaining a normal conversation difficult, but you're sure they'll notice something is wrong with you.

- Your senses seem dulled—food tastes bland and uninteresting, music doesn't seem to affect you, you don't bother smelling flowers anymore.

- The memory of every failure, every bad or uncomfortable experience, interview, or date comes into your mind incessantly and uncontrollably, like a torrent of negativity.

Listen to the Message of Depression

Somewhere in all the pain of depression, there has to be a message. Even when depression seems to come out of nowhere, it starts with a part of you signaling that something is not quite right. At the very least, it's a way of getting you to stop and think about your life—and possibly make some changes. It's all part of our human existence and God's alert system for our bodies, minds, emotions, and relationships, and we would be wise to heed these signals and warnings. It helps, therefore, to pause and ask yourself: "What is my depression telling me?"

For example, you may go into depression as you enter times of indecision. It may save you from impulsive decisions or actions that could have bad consequences. When you're at a significant crossroads in life, when your values and goals are shifting, and you're in a state of confusion, the angst and depression your mind creates could be keeping you in a period of indecision for a reason. It may be a call for careful evaluation and reflection.

Depression could also warn you of unresolved emotions, negative patterns of thinking, relationship conflicts, or chronic stress. It might appear after a time of God's blessing. Or, as discussed in the first chapter, it could be a sign of excessive strain and stress or being "stuck" and not knowing how to problem solve.

Whatever the message, however, it's important to heed it. Look at the feelings that come as warning signs and get help. Be proactive. Start caring for yourself right away. The longer you wait, the harder it will be.

Getting the Medical Care You Need

We've said before that you should get professional help as soon as possible. But if you feel you're depressed and your doctor is uninformed about depression in women, get a second opinion. Keep in mind, too, that some doctors will minimize health complaints in patients with a history of depression, even if the symptoms could be potentially serious.[2] If you are experiencing physical symptoms for which there is no clear explanation, see your doctor for an evaluation. If you have a history of medical or psychosomatic illnesses and believe that you have not had quality medical care, get another opinion. It may be that some other problem is being overlooked.

Patients who pay attention to detail and keep careful notes on what they observe about themselves can help their doctor tremendously. In addition:

- Talk honestly and openly about your symptoms, lifestyle, abusive behaviors, use of substances, and what is of concern to you. Try not to leave out anything. Remember, everything shared with a professional is confidential, and it is really important for determining the cause and treatment for your depression.
- Be specific when describing your symptoms. Don't just say, "I feel lousy and depressed." How is it affecting your sleep, appetite, sexuality, mood, concentration, and relationships?

- Ask questions of your doctor. Your questions will help your doctor communicate at an appropriate level. Think about your questions ahead of time and take a list of questions with you on your first visit to help you remember and keep to the point. If you don't understand any technical terms, options for treatment, requests for testing, or referrals to other doctors, ask for a simplified explanation at a level you can understand. (See Chapter 9 for additional guidance on what to ask your doctor regarding medications.)

- Take notes as you listen. Don't rely on your memory when you are depressed. This way you won't forget specifics of what you have learned at the appointment.

- Be your own health advocate. Remember, no one knows your body better than you. If something bothers you, if you want a particular test done, or you would like a referral for a second opinion, ask.

- If you don't feel that you can follow your doctor's advice, then say so. Be willing to partner with your doctor for your recovery. If you're not able to live with the possible side effects of a medication, ask if you could explore other options. Be sure you have a plan you can live with. Your compliance with the treatment program is crucial for overcoming and recovering from depression.

- Besides conventional treatment options such as counseling and medication, ask your doctor about natural complementary remedies and lifestyle changes you can make to prevent and reduce depression.

At this point you may be feeling a little overwhelmed by all the information we have provided. But don't be disheartened. In the chapters that follow, we'll guide you toward healing your pain. Take comfort in the fact that many have traveled this road ahead of you—and found a way out.

PART 2

Causes of Depression in Women

3

Depression Risk Factors

I will continue to praise you, God, even in my troubles and
   sufferings,
knowing that these afflictions will produce patient and
   unswerving endurance.
And this patience in turn develops maturity and
   character,
which produces joyful and confident hope of eternal
   salvation.
And that hope will never disappoint me.
For your love, God, has been poured out in my heart
through the Holy Spirit whom you have given to me.

Prayer inspired by Romans 5:5

Almost every woman has experienced suffering, loss,
pain, stress, disappointment, or illness. Frankly, it's part
of being human. But it's what happens next that makes
the difference. Though these experiences are common,
not every woman who goes through them develops clinical depression.

So what makes the depressed woman different? Hard to
say. It's also hard to say why some depressions appear out
of nowhere, with no real traumatic event as a catalyst.

The Muddy Fields of Cause and Comparison

By now, you know that there's not just one kind of depression—and there's not just one cause. In many respects, we were "designed" to become depressed under certain circumstances. Sometimes the depression is healthy, such as when it accompanies bereavement, but sometimes it is a symptom of a life gone wrong, as when chronic stress takes its toll. Research shows, in fact, that the causes of depression can be complex and multifaceted. In addition, because depression can impact every part of your being, problems in different areas of your life can make the clinical picture even muddier.

Let's not forget that personality factors also play a part, plus your physical makeup, body chemistry, the present quality of your marriage, how you were raised, your stage of life, and not least of all, the availability of nurturing people who understand your struggles and can go on loving you nonetheless. These factors all interact and overlap to make each depression distinct. While you have much in common with others when depressed, your depression is still uniquely yours. No one else on earth quite has the exact same depression.

In other words, don't compare yourself or your depression with others.

It's Not All in Your Head—Or Your Body

Trying to understand the origins of depression is in many ways similar to trying to understand the complexity of an illness like heart disease, diabetes, or cancer. Remember, depression is neither all in your head nor all in your body. It is not a sign of personal weakness nor is it a condition that you can overcome just by pulling yourself together.

Depression is the natural consequence of physical and situational factors.

So what's really behind the dramatic increase in women's depression? We know this much: Just as there are genetic factors that make some women more vulnerable to cancer or disease, there's a genetic factor for some women's depression.

Here, then, we're going to cover some of the "risk factors" for depression. Just as you can reduce your risk for heart disease by cutting out smoking, alcohol abuse, and overeating, there are things you can do to reduce your risk of depression. Unfortunately, the most obvious risk factor is being female—but let's focus on what we can change rather than what we can't.

The Calculated Risks

There are many factors that can predispose a woman to depression, and knowing what they are is the first step in prevention. Review the following and see if there are any themes with which you identify or current events that may become "triggers" for depression.

Psychosocial Risk Factors

First, let's look at risk factors in the psychosocial category, or those that arise from the psychological or social parts of our lives.

1. Early Developmental Struggles

Unresolved early developmental issues and childhood family dynamics can make a woman more susceptible to depression later in life. This is particularly so for the woman with a damaged sense of self. Critical and shaming parents can damage self-esteem and reduce a sense of self-mastery, also called self-efficacy. This leaves a woman with the belief that she is not as effective or efficacious in coping with the challenges of life. A simple task like dealing with a flat tire can seem overwhelming—and then make her depressed because she feels so incompetent.

When a sense of self isn't well developed and encouraged by parents in a positive way, a woman, when grown, can struggle with negative beliefs, distorted thinking patterns, and a lack of a sturdy sense of life. For these women, life will be more difficult.

A diminished sense of self is not the only childhood risk factor to be considered. We now know that many women, perhaps as many as 50 percent, have experienced some childhood loss or trauma, including inappropriate sexual touching or even abuse. These events can easily sensitize a woman emotionally, and if not resolved, can create a greater vulnerability to depression.

The journey to overcoming depression will need to include new, healthy, and encouraging relationships. Surround yourself with people who will walk with you as you relearn a healthy sense of self and self-sufficiency. A close relationship with God can be tremendously helpful, since the experience of God's deep love for you can often undo the damage done by a parent's neglect.

2. Mothers of Young Children

In our modern-day world, motherhood has a price. We strongly suspect that this wasn't so in previous ages, when women could focus on childbearing and not have to juggle as many roles as they do today. Being a woman with young children, therefore, is a risk factor to be considered. Childbearing women are very vulnerable to depression, and the more children a woman has, the more likely it is that she'll become depressed.

This fact is especially significant for stay-at-home moms to keep in mind. Those who have ill children, adolescents who act out, or few social outlets or outside interests of their own have a significantly increased risk. The risk for depression decreases, however, as these problems are dealt with.

3. Girls in Their Teens

Suicide is now the second leading cause of death from ages fifteen to nineteen, following only accidents. Young teens experience so many hormonal ups and downs that they have a more difficult time dealing with the stresses and challenges in their lives. For most teens, growing up is not all it's cracked up to be.

All relationships change as the prospect of adulthood approaches. Roles and expectations change dramatically almost by the year, and these can lead to deep emotional reactions. In addition, many of the teenage years involve saying good-bye to some things and embracing some others, and this can create many reactive depressions that overlay normal hormonally induced depressions. This is also the stage when we form our identity, confront the pressures of sexuality, begin to separate from parents, and make major, life-determining decisions.

We'll talk more about teen depression in the chapter on the woman's life cycle. Here, however, we want to stress how absolutely important it is to have a secure, loving, consistent, understanding, accepting home base. Teenagers who don't have such a home base and who don't feel connected to their friends and college community show a dramatic increase in risk for depression. *find a community – be intentional.*

4. The Pursuit of Thinness

Another explanation for why women get depressed more than men has to do with the current media emphasis on beauty being associated with being thin. Some women are discouraged with constantly dieting (unsuccessfully) to achieve the ideal cultural image, and this in turn has the devastating consequences of body image distortions, eating disorders, sexual inhibitions, and depression. Many studies confirm that developing adolescents are particularly vulnerable to being discontent with their changing bodies, resulting in depression.

5. Chronic Strain and Stress Response

Women tend to be under more chronic strain daily in and out of the home, and respond to stress differently than men. That could be another reason why they are at higher risk for depression. When under chronic strain and stress, women tend to feel powerless, helpless, and respond with behaviors such as ruminating. Dwelling on problems, negative thoughts, and emotions in turn feed the stress and it then becomes a vicious cycle. It drains women of motivation, persistence, and problem solving skills that could bring change. Refer to the chapter on stress, anxiety, and depression for more guidelines on this topic.

6. Baby Boomers and Other Generational Changes

Rates of clinical depression have increased in each succeeding generation since 1915 and are still rising. The greatest increases are being seen in teen girls.[1]

Recent studies suggest that the Baby Boomers of the post–World War II generation are particularly at risk for depression. Several explanations have been offered. The war certainly affected those who served in the armed forces, and many became parents afterwards. In addition, growing up in America during the 1950s and 1960s provided many emotional disruptions, including increased divorce rates and relocation that brought losses of family, friends, and community. Family life certainly changed during those years, and the sexual revolution didn't help. The children of that era are now aging, and there are more challenges facing them as the breakdown of the traditional nuclear family continues unabated.

7. Urban Dwellers

Major depression is more common in urban than in rural areas, but the difference doesn't hold true for other forms of depression, such as bipolar disorder. That could be because bipolar is generally regarded as having a stronger genetic cause. As for other depressions, we can only speculate why they're higher in urban areas. It's probably due to the stress impact of an urban-paced, hurried lifestyle. There's also greater disconnection and lack of community, which always increases the risk of depression.

So, if you live a fast-paced life in a major city, take precautions. Connect with a caring community; a church is probably the best community there is. Learn to slow down and build in recovery time. As someone once said, even if you win the "rat race," you'll still only be a rat—and probably a depressed one at that.

8. Poverty and Minority Status

Poverty can be a sure pathway to depression, and 75 percent of people living in poverty in the United States are women and children. Women who are ethnic minorities also experience great stress from discrimination. In addition, poor women often do not have access to basic mental health care, and this not only adds to their pressure and strain, but also means that their pain will last longer and be more disruptive to their already chaotic life pattern.

9. The Elderly

According to the National Depressive and Manic-Depressive Association, first episodes of depression usually occur in the early twenties to thirties, but it's not uncommon for them to appear later in life. As more and more people live longer lives, an increase in depression among the elderly is expected. An aging body is simply not as resilient as a young body and will experience a greater incidence of biochemical breakdown.

Many factors contribute to increased risk of depression among the elderly. Chronic illness takes its toll on brain chemistry. Major changes in lifestyle—such as forced retirement or the loss of a husband, which is common for women in their sixties and seventies—will make women more prone to reactive depressions. Also, elderly women face an increased frequency of the death of friends and family, and it is disconnecting and depressing to be the last one left. Many elderly just give up the will to live, and without such a will, there's little to protect them from depression.

Despite the increase in risk for depression as we age, there is still some good news. Regardless of age or cause, depression can be treated. Many elderly women, therefore, need to be encouraged to seek treatment, so that whatever life remains for them can be of the highest quality possible.

10. Other Psychosocial Risk Factors

So far, the risk factors mentioned are pretty common. Other factors affect fewer women, but they're still important. They include alcohol abuse and addictions to drugs or sex. Sexual addiction is usually considered a male problem, but some women are at risk here also. Women with these conditions need to get help right away, not just for depression, but for underlying addictions that may serve to self-medicate their despondency.

Biological Risk Factors

Biological risk factors make up the second major group of issues in the lives of most women. This is where we see the greatest difference between genders. Male depression is much less affected by hormonal or other biological factors than women's.

1. Imbalances of Brain Chemical Messengers

Neurochemicals, which drive our brain's activities, can best be understood as "messengers." Basically, they're the brain's communication system. Some of these neurotransmitters are happy messengers, and some are sad messengers. (There's a more detailed description of these messengers in Dr. Hart's book, *The Anxiety Cure.*) If you're seriously depressed, you can pretty much assume that your messenger system's biochemistry is upset.

High levels of the stress hormone cortisol block an important tranquilizing messenger called "GABA," and the result is a state of increased anxiety. This, in turn, increases your risk for depression. Other mechanisms also disturb depression-related messengers such as serotonin, and this also increases your risk for depression. Women tend to have lower serotonin levels than men. We'll cover more on that later.

2. Family History of Depression

A family history of depression is a strong marker for depression; in other words, it increases your risk. Those with close family members who have been depressed are about twice as likely as the average person to become seriously depressed themselves. Close female relatives of depressed women have a one in four chance of depression and a 90 percent chance of having mild depression. Relatives who are a little more distant from depressed people, such as cousins, uncles, or aunts, have a 15 percent chance of inheriting major depression.

This could be due to genetics or to family relationships and socialization. Some families have an inherited genetic vulnerability to depression, particularly in the case of bipolar disorders, where up to 50 percent of manic-depressives have at least one parent with the disorder. Researches have concluded that we don't inherit depression solely as a result of one gene, like hair or eye color, but possibly several genes. Depression can be attributed to only about a 40 percent influence by genes. Certain personality traits collectively known as depressive personality disorder, however, may make a woman more prone to depression.[2]

3. Reproductive Hormones

If there is one biological factor that truly separates the sexes, it's the roles of reproduction. Men clearly have it easier here, since all the risk lies with women.

Depression can clearly be linked to the mood-altering hormonal effects of the reproductive cycle. Every aspect of reproduction, including menstruation, pregnancy, childbirth, and the use of oral contraceptives, can be linked to an increased risk for depression. The dramatic changes in psychoactive hormones like estrogen and progesterone that occur during menstrual cycles and during pregnancy are believed to be key factors in affecting mood-regulating transmitters. The estrogen/progesterone dance can cause a range of problems, from the monthly blues to an ongoing cycle of depression over a longer period of time. Miscarriage, infertility, and surgical menopause can also cause depressive symptoms. We will discuss this in more detail in the chapter on the life cycle of women.

4. Hormonal Drugs and Medications

Hormonal drugs such as birth control pills and steroids such as cortisone and prednisone may also cause depression. In addition, medications for problems such as high blood pressure and arthritis can cause depression as a side effect. If you're on medication for a physical problem, check with your doctor about possible side effects and discuss all types and dosages of medications you're on.

5. Medical Conditions

Depression is common with a number of medical conditions. The list includes: endocrine disorders such as thyroid problems, heart disease, heart attacks, recovery from open-heart surgery, cancer, recovery from stroke, and other disorders such as anxiety, addictions, eating disorders, and substance abuse. If the depression accompanying a medical condition goes untreated, it could actually worsen the medical disorder and hinder its treatment.

6. Chronic Illness, Disability, and Coexistent Illness

Depression is often secondary to other conditions; this is called comorbidity, since two disorders coexist. For example, women with panic disorder, obsessive compulsive disorder, generalized anxiety disorder, post traumatic stress disorder, an eating disorder, or a personality disorder are at high risk for a comorbid clinical depression, which is frequently unrecognized and therefore untreated.

Substance abuse disorders often coexist with depression. Sometimes the substance is used to self-medicate depression, but then becomes a problem in its own right. Once the substance use has been discontinued, additional treatment will be necessary if the depression still persists.

Depression can act as a cover for many other illnesses, and this fact is often overlooked. For example, a recent study suggests that as many as thirteen million Americans may be unaware that they have endocrine disorders such as hypothyroidism (an underactive thyroid gland) or hyperthyroidism (overactive thyroid gland). When the thyroid pumps too much or too little, it causes nervous-

Biochemical and Physiological Causes of Depression

There are many medical and physiological factors that can cause depression. Following are some of the underlying factors that can cause or contribute to depression in women. If you suspect that you have any of these disorders together with depression, talk to your doctor:

Allergies, both atmospheric and food sources

Alzheimer's disease

Candidiasis, or chronic overgrowth of yeast in the gut

Chronic inflammation

Chronic pain, including ongoing physical or emotional pain

Drug abuse, including prescription, illicit, alcohol, caffeine, and nicotine

Head trauma

Hormonal imbalances such as PMS, perimenopause, or endocrine gland difficulties

Hypoglycemia; low blood sugar can lead to chronic mood swings and depression

Hypothyroidism; low levels of thyroid hormone can lead to exhaustion and depression

Infectious diseases; problems such as strep throat affect the immune system

Intestinal parasites; symptoms of parasitic infection include brain fog, depression, and feelings of doom

Lack of exercise; those who don't exercise are three times as likely to be depressed

Nutritional deficiencies or excesses, such as insufficiency of omega–3 oils, Vitamin B-complex, Vitamin C, iron, calcium, magnesium, or potassium

Major illnesses such as diabetes, cancer, a brain tumor, or disease of the heart, lung, or liver

Multiple sclerosis

Parkinson's disease

Rheumatoid arthritis

Seasonal affective disorder (SAD)

Seizure-related conditions

Sleep disorders

Stress/low adrenal function, such as low levels of serotonin and norepinephrine

Stroke

ness or depression, weight loss or gain, bursts of energy or exhaustion. If untreated, it can lead to other serious physical problems.

Relationship Risk Factors

Many risk factors for female depression can be found in the social environment and in the quality or absence of meaningful relationships. Women tend to be more people-oriented than men. This can bring a lot of fulfillment and satisfaction in life, but it also means that women are more vulnerable to depression from relationship loss, strain, conflict, and unresolved issues.[3] Women are also more vulnerable to victimization and abuse by men. Following are some ways women are socially and relationally at risk for depression:

1. Sexual and Physical Abuse

The American Psychological Association's Task Force on Women and Depression reports that 37 percent of depressed women have suffered significant physical or sexual abuse by age twenty-one. Some experts actually believe that the rate may be closer to 50 percent. Violent episodes such as battering and rape may leave women with post traumatic stress disorder, with depression as the consequence. Also, undiagnosed head trauma from battering may cause depressive symptoms because of the damage to the brain. Abuse may lead to low self-esteem, a sense of helplessness, self-blame, and social isolation, and these can all be the cause of depression.

2. Marriage and Children

Married women have higher rates of depression than unmarried women. In unhappy marriages, women are three times as likely as men to be depressed. Mothers of young children are very vulnerable to depressive symptoms, and the more children a woman has, the more likely it is that she'll be depressed.

3. Social and Role Pressures

Women are usually caring for and supporting others such as children, husbands, and sometimes aging parents. Additional multiple role changes are taking place for women. They are increasingly assuming leadership positions in government, industry, business, and even the church. More and more women are becoming the primary breadwinners of their families or having to financially contribute by working outside the home. And with the increasing cost of living and rising incidence of divorce, women are facing dramatic changes in their daily stress load and complexity of roles, which can all increase the risk of depression.

4. Low Self-esteem

Diminished self-esteem can cause depression, or it can be caused by depression. Women seem to experience challenges to their self-esteem more often than men. Lowered self-esteem can be due to a variety of personal, relational, and cultural issues. For instance, being sensitive to what others think, being torn about whom to please, and feeling blamed or blaming yourself for relationship failures can all damage self-esteem. Unresolved identity confusion and unclear life goals can also add to the problem.

When women stay at home and raise small children, they may feel that others around them don't value their role or contribution to society. Unfortunately, our success-driven culture emphasizes work and career building above everything else—especially the mundane task of being a mother—and this can have subtle effects on a woman's sense of value. The truth is, however, that there can be no greater privilege than to raise children.

5. Singleness and Single Parenting

Results from several U.S. and Canadian surveys presented at the May 2000 annual meeting of the American Psychiatry Association in Chicago suggest that at any given time, single moms are nearly twice as likely to be depressed as married moms. This is not surprising, since there is no doubt in our minds that single moms have a much more challenging job before them. They have to raise children alone. They are the primary financial providers. Caregiving always results in chronic stress, but being the sole responsible parent significantly increases the strain of financial pressures and child-care resources. Balancing work, parenting, self-care, and meaningful connections with other people can cause a woman to be at risk for depression.

6. Attachment Losses

Because women tend to be more emotionally connected, having the primary care role in the family, they are at greater risk for loss-related depressions.

As we mentioned earlier, because women tend to be more relational, they also tend to develop more intimate bonds with their friends and family. This puts them at greater risk for depression whenever there are changes to—and losses of—relationships. In the next chapter, we'll deal specifically with depression that comes from loss. Loss needs to be grieved, and the better able we are to do our grieving, the greater our chances for healing.

Mental and Cognitive Risk Factors

Cognitive and thinking patterns can also be the basis of depressions that are unique to women.

1. Personality Styles and Psychological Makeup

Some women have a lower personal threshold and a vulnerability to becoming more easily depressed than others. Women who are more passive and dependent on others, who are pessimistic, and who feel they have little control over life events are more easily overwhelmed with stress and more likely to be vulnerable to depression—particularly if they dwell on their low feelings. Melancholic personality types also tend to be prone to depression, due to their deep capacity for feeling and sometimes pessimistic outlook. Creative, artistic, expressive people like painters, writers, musicians, and actors have higher rates of depression, too.

2. Learned Helplessness or No Sense of Control

Feelings of helplessness can lead to depression. In a sense, helplessness is a loss of control, and loss leads to depression. Feelings of helplessness can be quite serious—and common—in women. That's because much of our present-day world is geared toward men. Women can easily come to feel that they are out of control and have little power to change this.

Much research has gone into understanding this phenomenon, and what has emerged is something called "learned helplessness." In other words, feelings of helplessness don't just appear out of the blue; they're learned, usually from a young age. Once you believe that there is nothing you can do to change your circumstances, helplessness becomes hopelessness—and then depression.

Whatever the origin, helplessness can be unlearned and replaced with new beliefs, skills, and patterns. With some therapeutic help, you can learn how to avoid helpless feelings and thus build a resistance to depression.

3. Rumination

One of the main differences between men and women is the way they respond to stress and trouble. Women tend

Risk Factors for Depression

Read through the following list and mark those that apply to you. Take this list with you to your doctor and/or psychotherapist, so that he or she can see the whole picture as a treatment plan is developed. Remember, men, this list applies only to women.

Pain/challenges in your life
__Frustration over several life issues
__Disappointment/feelings of helplessness and hopelessness
__Conflicts in marriage
__Conflicts over children
__Dealing with difficult people/relationships
__Parenting struggles; burden over being a mom and raising children correctly
__Keeping a proper balance/priorities in all areas of your life
__Juggling roles with family and outside interests/vocations
__Role overload; getting bogged down in the mundane
__Knowing who you are, your destiny, calling, and contribution on earth, and feeling fulfilled
__The angst of being transformed or becoming whole
__Battling the same old issues, such as family stuff, weaknesses, character traits, and defenses
__Battling overwhelming emotions such as anger, disillusion, loneliness, fear, or disappointment
__Unexpected change or loss
__Intense periods of focusing on one area of life
__Neglecting to care for and nurture yourself
__Not living a balanced life, such as having young children at home, going to school, working full time, and still having to keep up with household duties
__Being physically ill or having a loved one who is ill
__Not having a place to call "home"
__Not being able to have children
__Not having enough money

Past traumas
__Early losses
__Dysfunctional patterns that were learned or experienced in family of origin
__Abuse, including physical, sexual, or emotional
__Neglect and abandonment

continued

__Traumatic life events
__Domestic violence

Reactions to life circumstances
__Guilt of sin
__Indecision
__Anger
__Bitterness
__Unforgiveness
__Times of transition and change
__Stress and strain
__Disappointment, loss, or bereavement
__Sadness
__Unrealistic expectations
__Hormonal life cycle changes
__Marriage and parenting strain
__Being a stay-at-home mom

Continuous struggles
__Chronic disappointment
__Chronic illness such as cancer or heart disease
__Chronic stress
__Abusive relationships
__Financial problems or poverty
__Distorted body image
__Cultural pressures for the pursuit of thinness
__Eating disorders
__Lack of meaning in life
__Low self-esteem
__Unresolved identity as a woman
__Role overload in caring for others
__Role confusion in not knowing how to be fulfilled
__Negative patterns of thinking (rumination)
__Learned helplessness or no sense of control
__Chronic indecision/poor decision making skills
__Unexpressed and/or unresolved emotions
__Patterns of vulnerability to risk factors of recurring depression
__Genetic predisposition
__Hormone imbalances and fluctuations such as PMS or postpartum
   issues

to act "inwardly," think, and ruminate over a problem situation. This usually results in pessimistic thinking and negative emotions. Men, on the other hand, tend to act "outwardly," and by taking action, cut off the depression.

What You Can Do

Hopefully, this chapter has opened your eyes to the many things that can increase your chances of depression. Our purpose is not to overwhelm you, but to help you gain a stronger sense of control over your depression. The more you know about your problem, the more empowered you'll be to deal with it.

None of the risk factors we have described are insurmountable. Every one can be challenged and overcome. If you're depressed, it's very likely that you don't feel very empowered right now. But take heart; by the time you finish this book, we believe you'll feel a greater sense of control.

At this point, all that's required is that you keep reading. Follow the suggestions we offer and don't be troubled by how hard it may seem or whether you fail to do it right. Just start over when you have to. If it's too hard to do it alone, reach out to a friend, pastor, or professional counselor for help. This is not a sign of weakness. On the contrary, our experience has been that it's the strongest people who have the courage to reach out for help, not the weakest.

Above all, continue to remain in a spirit of prayer. Lean as hard as you can on God for his empowerment in your life. As it says in Psalm 23, he has promised to walk with us through life's darkest moments, and he has never failed to keep that promise.

4

Loss and Depression

Spirit of God, comfort me as I mourn;
give me beauty instead of ashes, the oil of joy for mourn-
     ing, the garment of praise instead of a heavy, burdened
     and failing spirit.
So that I may be called a strong tree of righteousness,
the planting of you, Lord, and that you may be glorified.

Prayer inspired by Isaiah 61:3

all forms

Loss is inevitable, and continuing to live after a major life loss takes courage, strength that we sometimes fear we don't have, and support from the shelter that only those who care about us can provide.

Let's look at the case of Gerald Sittser, who lost his mother, wife, and daughter one night in a car accident. Out of his experience, he says that the defining moments of our lives are made up of the way we respond to our losses. These responses shape the quality and direction of our lives.

Granted, you don't have to lose a mother, wife, or child to feel the deep pain of loss, sadness, or depression. It may be the loss of a dream, a relationship, or even the realization that life hasn't turned out as you expected.

What are we called to do when life dishes up a significant loss? First, we need to grieve that loss, no matter how small or big it is. This is how God has designed us. If the object or person we have lost is important to us, then it, he, or she is important enough to be grieved. Whatever your life holds for you, when a major loss comes your way, whether it is important or not, expected or unexpected, necessary or unnecessary, you should be prepared to deal with the loss through the process of grieving. It will take time, and may be extremely painful, but there is no other way to the other side, where you'll learn to live without that loss.

This is Dr. Hart here, and I remember giving that same advice to my middle daughter, Sharon Hart Morris. Here's her story:

> Losses. We've all felt them. I have. I have lost dreams, lost my way, lost opportunities, sometimes lost hope, and at times, even lost the sense of where God was leading me. But my most painful loss was the death of my husband when he was only thirty-five years old. It was my most feared loss. Those times were the worst of times. Sometimes I cried until I fell asleep, and other times tears just couldn't come. Showering was exhausting. Afternoons were spent curled on a couch, staring at nothing. Boiling water seemed a complicated task. Everything was a haze, like walking through a fog. Stunned by the shock, my senses were so stimulated that they were used up feeling the shock and left me in a daze. The simplest tasks seemed difficult and impossible to do. There was no desire, nor energy left to reach out to others. I remember driving with my father to the church to make funeral arrangements. "Daddy," I asked him, "how long will it take for it to not hurt so much?" "Oh," answered my dear daddy, "it takes a while, and if there are complications, it takes longer. But the only way to the other side, dear Sharon, is through it."

When Loss Leads to Depression

As we said earlier, the treatment of a particular depression depends a lot on the cause of the depression. We will once again, then, make distinction between situational-based depressions and biological-based depressions. This chapter will focus on situational or reactive depressions; those brought on by what happens in the external world. The best understood and most severe form of reactive depression we, as humans, can experience is that of bereavement. There is no greater loss than the death of someone you love very much. But painful as the grief of death can be, *all* other losses in life have to be dealt with through the same grieving process. The only difference between the loss of bereavement and, say, the loss of being dismissed from your job, is one of severity.

Life's Losses

Any meaningful loss has the potential to trigger depression. In general, the more meaningful the loss, the greater the depression.

The potential for loss starts early, as soon as we're born, and we lose the safety and comfort of the womb. And as we grow, that potential for loss increases by the day. We "lose" our mother's breast when we're old enough to eat regular food. We "lose" the safety of home when we start kindergarten. We get slighted by friends on the playground, we get a failing grade in class, our bike gets stolen, or we don't get that cherished part in the school play. Later, friends move away, we don't get into the college of our choice, or a potential romantic relationship doesn't work out. And that's just for starters. Then come the real losses, the potential life challenges of a failed marriage, divorce, a friend's cancer, a partner's serious illness, infertility, infidelity, and finally death itself.

As you can see, we can't escape loss in life. It's there in the shadows from the first breath to the last, and in every stage of life, we must let go of what's behind so we can embrace what's ahead. Loss is there when we transition from adolescence to adulthood, taking responsibility for earning a living. Loss is there again as soon as we've earned a little money and try to make a risky investment. It is especially there when we think about getting married, and we trade the loss of freedom for the hope of intimacy and companionship. Eventually, we begin to lose our faculties as well, such as memory, teeth, and eyesight.

For some, life seems to dish out a disproportionate amount of painful experiences, and all of them involve some aspect of loss. These people seem to face disaster at every turn. More loved ones die early, more children go off the rails, and more illnesses seem to strike than in the average home. If you have experienced these losses we pray that, in some way, God will comfort you and turn your excessive pain into a glorious blessing.

Loss is even addressed in the Bible. The writer of the book of Ecclesiastes, possibly King Solomon, describes what it feels like to suffer in this way. In Chapter 2, verses 17 and 18, he gives a perfect description of the feelings of depression and despair when he writes:

> So I hated life, because the work that is done under the sun was grievous to me. All of it is meaningless, a chasing after the wind. I hated all the things I had toiled for under the sun, because I must leave them to the one who comes after me.

And then in Chapter 3, verses 1 to 8, he gives us that beautiful and comforting summary of life, including its necessary grieving experiences:

> There is a time for everything, . . . a time to be born, and a time to die, . . . a time to weep and a time to laugh, a time to mourn and a time to dance.

There is no greater wisdom than this. Life is all about loss. Some of it is necessary, because if we don't let go, we can't embrace what lies ahead, but a whole lot of it is unnecessary loss that we could have avoided. Regardless, the loss must be grieved. And through the depression it brings, it will mature us. That's the way we were made.

Loss = Anxiety + Depression

Overall, life can seem disappointing and very unfair. If you love someone dearly, you will eventually have to let that person go, and it's going to hurt. You can avoid such hurt by never loving anyone, but that doesn't seem like a good solution to this dilemma of life. Our world has been designed in such a way that loss is inevitable, and that to usher in the new, the old must be surrendered. This is how God ordained it. We either learn how to deal with loss in a positive way, or we experience the inevitable melancholy or depression.

But just how does loss become anxiety and depression? Judith Viorst describes it well:

> Loss gives rise to anxiety when the loss is either impending or thought to be temporary. Anxiety contains a kernel of hope. But when loss appears to be permanent, anxiety (protest) gives way to depression (despair).[1]

In addition to feeling lonely and sad, we may also feel that we are responsible for driving the person away or feel helpless in that there's nothing we can do to bring the person back. We may also feel unlovable or hopeless, that we'll be this way forever.

Was That Really Necessary?

We've already talked about life's necessary losses, the ones that are simply part of life, part of releasing the past and embracing the future. There's also a category of loss considered "unnecessary." For example, you may have been warned about hanging out with "no-good" guys while you were a teenager, but because they made you feel desirable, you got yourself into trouble. Or maybe, to avoid pain, you started using substances that you've become addicted to. Or one step further, maybe you've realized that you should have received that education, had children, or taken advantage of other opportunities while you still had the chance.

Each of these losses could have been avoided, but because of negligence, ignorance, or rebellion, we have all made some bad choices—and now live with the consequences. You're not alone. All of us have had our fair share of these losses. You could say, actually, that they're necessary, too—necessary for making us learn and mature.

Maybe God Designed Us for Depression

At first glance, this doesn't seem to make sense. Why would a loving God intentionally allow us to go through such painful experiences? But God knew, when he created us as finite beings, locked into time with an end in view, how much we would have to struggle with the losses that go along with finiteness. So he wisely made provision for this in the healing power of grief. The purposeful nature and importance of grief is one of the most transforming discoveries I, Dr. Hart, have ever made. And it didn't come from my study of psychology. It came from my understanding of life, informed by Scripture.

I began my clinical career really baffled by how devastating depression could be for people. For a long time, I struggled to reconcile this painful malady with a loving God. Often, while trying to help someone in a deep, demoralizing depression, I would ask myself the question,

"Why does God allow such pain into our lives?" Needless to say, we have no clear answers to such questions. We refer to dilemmas like this as mysteries, but it doesn't really help.

Then it suddenly dawned on me that God had actually designed us to become depressed under certain conditions.

Now I know that in times of deep depression, it's hard to see any purpose lurking behind our despair and darkness. However, we need to hold on to the belief that despite the pain, there is a good outcome ahead. Depression helps us release that which we have lost. So the real problem is not our depression but that, given the way life works, sooner or later something or someone must leave us. Nothing lasts forever, at least not this side of eternity. If we want to achieve a satisfying—even happy—life, all we have to do is cooperate with the process God has provided us. So King Solomon is correct in that there is nothing new under the sun, there is "a time to weep . . . and a time to mourn." If we do our weeping and mourning, then there will be "a time to laugh . . . and a time to dance."

Women's Necessary Losses

There are many "necessary" losses in every woman's life, and it will be helpful to review them here. That way, you can be assured you're not crazy or all alone in your experience. Life presents all of us with losses, but some are unique to women. Anticipating these losses ahead of time can help you prepare; even necessary losses can be devastating when they catch us by surprise.

1. Losses Can Start in Early Childhood

The most important loss a child can experience is that of a parent or sibling through death or separation. Relationship losses in the early, vulnerable stages of childhood development account for most of the first episodes of depression in a child's life. Those who are depressed report a much higher incidence of having lost a parent in childhood than among other people.[2] For most women, this early loss is a "father loss." Such a loss could be due to death, divorce, neglect, or abandonment. The loss of a brother or sister early in life can also precipitate depression in girls and influence later depressions. Because divorce is so common these days, it is not uncommon for children to lose siblings when a family is split. Such early losses can condition you to distrust or fear potential relationship losses later in life.

2. Moving On Means Letting Go

Through the seasons and passages of adult life, each stage brings challenges of both change and growth. Every woman's journey is going to be unique to her circumstances, development, and opportunities, but it still may be helpful to see the overall life journey as a series of seasons. This is important to help your perspective in the larger scope of life.

Early Adulthood (18 to 30)

Here we lose the protective covering of childhood and awaken to the responsibilities, worries, and wonder of adulthood. In our twenties, we search for meaning, purpose, and our place in the world. Many of us seek out a major in college, exploring our newfound freedom and wings. We search for our first real job. Some of us venture into marriage. Then, children may enter our lives. For some, we learn how to juggle a career, husband, and children, and for others, the search for that one special man continues. This can be disappointing, lonely, and filled with questions of why God fills us with the deep longing for love, but frustrates us in making us wait until a husband is found.

First Adulthood (30 to 45)

These years are filled with adventure. One adventure is being "married with children." Here, children consume our time and energy. Marriage is hard work. And hopes for a career are either put on hold or squeezed into a hectic schedule of kids, husband, and home responsibilities.

For some women, marriage is torn apart, which ushers in new seasons of single parenting and singleness. A second marriage, with a whole new set of stepchildren, may enter your life. This is an adventure, too, because blended families are even harder work. And yet, life urges us forward, refining, challenging, and forcing us to look at who we are, how we interact, and how we live our lives. For those who don't marry, coming to terms with singleness—or the continued dream and hope of a married life—continues. Heartaches, new friendships, and new adventures open up that otherwise would not have. All the while, we trust that God does have a future for us, one with hope, purpose, and love.

Second Adulthood (45 to 85+)

This season is filled with transitions, losses, and a renewed outlook on life. Kids grow up and (maybe) leave home for college or marriage. At forty-five or fifty, we may find ourselves with an empty house, perimenopausal symptoms, and a whole new era of life ahead of us. Should we start a new career, go back to school, pick up long-lost hobbies, travel, or embark on an adventure that is new, scary, and wonderful? Yes, even at seventy years of age, life still awaits us. Relationships are richer, maturity has settled in, and with the wisdom of age and the experience of time, we are able to move more purposefully and gracefully through the golden years.

Yet, it is all mixed with losses. Sometimes marriage fails. Hair turns gray and begins to thin out. Wrinkles appear out of nowhere, bulges cling like long-lost friends, and our once energetic bodies begin to slow down and even fail. We write our lists of things that we will never do, mourn those losses, and then write a new list of what we can do with the life we have left. Friends become ill, some die, and the shortness of life becomes a sharp reality. Slowly it dawns on us that we don't live forever. We won't always have a tomorrow. Our children, friends, and loved ones won't always be available for a cup of tea or a shopping spree. Life eventually and inevitably comes to an end. Those who are most fortunate are able to sit on the porch of old age and rock back and forth, savoring their yesterdays, enjoying the sacred moment of the now, eagerly awaiting the words, "welcome home, my good and faithful servant."

3. The Family Life Cycle Can Bring Loss

As parents, we raise young people who need to be nurtured, protected, loved, cared for, taught, guided, and equipped. We spend (at least) eighteen years doing this, so that one day they can leave and be responsible, capable, beautiful, loving human beings, who are able to develop and thrive in healthy relationships—but away from us. Parenting, therefore, is fraught with losses and grieving.

4. You Can Lose Identity and Self-esteem

Women generally flourish in relationships. Usually, self-worth is found not so much in accomplishing great things, but rather in contributing to the lives of others and to society as a whole.

The demands of our many roles and the fast-paced lifestyle force us to negotiate a meaningful and purposeful life that doesn't really fit our deepest needs. We want to garden, read, build friendships, raise a family, go back to school, or even write a book, but it all takes time, energy, and focus, and competes with the many other demands already upon us.

Our self-esteem and sense of worth depend on our ability to prioritize and balance our deep personal aspirations along with the demands of family and work. As women, we often place ourselves, our dreams, and our desires on the back burner while the needs of others take priority.

All of this is to say that identity, self-worth, and self-esteem are very fragile in the life of women today. Much has changed and is changing, but no longer can women rely only on their competence as mothers and homemakers for their sense of value.

5. Dreams Can Go Unfulfilled

For women, more so than men, dreams can be the first casualty of life. And this can easily lead to depression.

Are women more prone to being dreamers? Possibly. Nothing much happens without a dream. As women, we're filled with longings, dreams, and desires from our earliest years. Playing with dolls helped us to dream about being mothers one day. And as more and more career opportunities opened up to us, we also dreamed about becoming lawyers and doctors. But dreams aren't always fulfilled. Life can be disappointing and fail to deliver what we had expected. Some of us dreamed of being married and settling down with our own family. We dreamed of raising children—and then found we couldn't have them. Others of us hoped to celebrate a 50th wedding anniversary with our childhood sweethearts—but divorce or death got in the way.

Many married women have had to put their dreams on hold to stay home and care for children and discover that they're way behind when they reenter the marketplace. Some have even found themselves redundant. This is Dr. Weber speaking. My sister Sylvia is a singer and a praise and worship leader. She would love to express her talents in concert halls, yet she expresses her gifts primarily in her local church community. She chose to place her desire to sing full-time and travel extensively on the back burner to raise her three children. One day, during a painful season in her life, she wrote a song. That very song was chosen as the theme song for the Focus on the Family women's conferences. During the yearlong conferences, over 300,000 women across the nation sang her song, and Sylvia rejoiced. Yes, she sings like a songbird to her children every night as she puts them to bed, and no other audience could ever compare. But the experience taught her that God did not forget the longings of her heart. He placed them there, after all. He sees what we long to do, to know, and to accomplish. And even if our dreams are delayed, detoured, or never come about the way we want, we can still hold on to the faithfulness of God.

Remember: You're only in one season of life at a time, and it, too, will pass. Bloom where you're planted. Hold the seeds that can only be planted in the spring when all signs of frost are gone. Wait. Plant them then. Soon, spring will come. Be patient. Enjoy today, because that's what God has given you to live with now.

6. You May Feel You're Not Being Good Enough

Many married women are not so concerned about success and failure as they are about being a good enough

mother or homemaker—making their life count for something by doing things that are useful and meaningful for
others. In addition, career women are faced with a huge
challenge fraught with potential for losses, namely, being
successful in the working world.

It's well known in stress research that the ratio of success to failure can determine the rate of burnout and
depression in both men and women. When a sense of failure is experienced more than success, there is a greater
risk of developing a reactive depression. A person who has
had a long history of failures is more prone to depression
and will experience that depression more deeply when
confronted with a significant life loss.

So, what's the "right" way to deal with failure? First, we
must look at God's view on success and failure. God is less
concerned about our success than he is with who we are
"becoming." Success, by the world's standards, never builds
character, nor does it make us better people in God's eyes.

Also, in God's view, every failure is an opportunity for
growth. Someone once said, "Success is built upon a
mountain of failures." If this is true, and we believe it is,
then why do we fear failure as much as we do? Finally,
success in God's eyes has a lot to do with faithfulness, not
winning. This is very clear from the parable of the talents,
in which God praises the servants who did what they were
told to do. "Well done, good and faithful servant," he says
in Matthew 25:21. God's prize doesn't go to the winner of
the race, but to the one who finishes the race. This means
that we all can win. It also means that, to be successful in
God's eyes, we only have to be obedient.

7. Your "Life's Work" May Be Unfulfilling

Both men and women can be disillusioned with their
life's work. From doctors to seamstresses, from business

executives to janitors, most people come to realize that their work, exciting as it may have been to start with, sooner or later becomes unfulfilling and unsatisfying. And this can result in depression.

Women are actually at greater risk for becoming depressed over work than men. Some women are working demanding, unfulfilling jobs because they weren't able to get training or higher education and were forced into the workplace out of financial necessity. Women are also still up against tremendous obstacles to progress in the workplace. In some arenas, the working world still favors men. In general, men find it easier to fit themselves into a career. In addition, women with families need more flexible work hours, child care options, medical benefits, and the like. Whatever the reason, however, the challenges facing women today as they try to find their place in the working world are still great— and fraught with disappointment, frustration, stress, despair, and depression.

8. Marriage Isn't Always the "Safe Haven" You Imagined

One of the messages we fail to teach young people is just how hard it is to build a fulfilling, happy marriage. We happen to believe that the best chance for doing this is when both partners are committed Christians. But even then, it takes hard work. Failure to make your marriage a safe haven where both partners feel emotionally secure and supported is bound to be cause for reactive depressions.

Illness, severe emotional disorder in your partner, the consequences of childhood trauma, and many other factors can undermine the security and happiness of a marriage and impose a severe strain on everyone involved. Obviously, there's a lot women can do to improve their marriages. But our culture has reinforced the belief that a good marriage just happens, and if it doesn't, you should simply cut your losses and move on to the next partner. After all, that's what we see in the movies.

If you don't believe you can trust your partner or that he is available and responsive to your needs, then we strongly recommend that you seek help from a competent marriage counselor. If your partner won't go with you, go alone. It's amazing what a counselor can do to help a marriage just by working with one partner. So take care of yourself, and in so doing, you might be able to impact your partner to do the same.

9. Children Can Disappoint You

Most married couples can't imagine what life would be like without children. And as our children grow, we begin to anticipate their self-development. Our dreams for them may sometimes reach beyond the stars and need to be brought back to reality, but by the time our children become teenagers, we've begun to accept their limits— though still hoping that they will be successful and live fulfilling, happy lives.

But what if that doesn't happen? What if some disaster befalls them? What if they get caught up in drugs or fall into the wrong crowd and end up in some serious trouble? It happens, even in the best of circles. I've seen good parents become totally shattered by a wayward kid, a child who completely goes off the rails. When this happens, all your dreams for them are shattered. Your own life seems a total waste in the light of such disappointment. And this is a lot more common than you might think.

What can parents do when children disappoint? Obviously, continue to love them and pray for them. Then let your children go. Release them into God's hands. Leave the matter with God.

In the Pit

We've already stated that all losses must be grieved, whether they were necessary or unnecessary losses. If this grieving is not done properly, reactive depression will be the result. And do not underestimate the power of reactive depression to affect your life. Many suicides are not just the result of serious biological depressions; they're from severe reactive depressions as well. This is Dr. Hart again, and I've done quite a bit of bereavement psychotherapy. One of the greatest challenges to the therapist is to reinstill the will to live.

Physical symptoms of reactive depression such as lethargy and excessive sleep may not be as disruptive as those of other depressions, but the sadness can reach far deeper into the psyche and have a longer impact. You may feel as though you are damned, even rejected, by God. Your friends may try to comfort you, but your emotional ears are deaf to their reassurances. You feel what you feel, no matter what they say. You feel terribly frightened, but your friends keep insisting everything is going to be okay. Fear permeates every aspect of your life, undermining your confidence. You can't make the smallest decisions.

In reactive depression, you can feel quite guilty, especially if you feel responsible for the loss you have suffered. Rational thinking is difficult. Often you feel that your brain has shut down because you can't think. Even though you feel a profound sadness, your mind seems to be numb to all other emotions. Every action, every thought, is a cause for anxiety. You feel like a failure and you beg for forgiveness. You want to keep punishing yourself, hoping you will get rid of the terrible feelings inside. You remem-

ber bad things you did when you were a child and wish
you could go back and make amends. Often, you will wake
up in the morning feeling as if everything is right again.
Then you remember, and the sense of loss associated with
your depression returns again to haunt you through the
rest of the day.

For some, the feelings are mild and they move on rapidly. For others, it just takes time—lots of time. And for
still others, it's a deep pain that never seems to let up. Every
one of these losses must be grieved if you are to restore a
sense of hope and happiness again.

Take It to the Cross

As Christians, we're uniquely equipped to deal with
reactive depression. Not only does our faith provide the
resources of the Holy Spirit to help us come to terms with
the loss, but the gospel also gives us insight into one of
life's major problems: the fact that life is transitory. Eventually we lose everything on this earth, including life itself.

Human nature is remarkably tenacious. For reasons of
security, fear, or comfort, we don't let go very easily. When
we love, we also want to possess; when we want something we desire, it becomes an obsession. Powerful forces
attract us to what we own. Because we cling to posses-
sions, ideas, reputations, and people, we experience losses
very deeply, and the ensuing depression is unnecessarily
painful and prolonged. The problem of depression is not
the loss; it is the attachment to the lost object. We have to
learn to let it go.

This is one of the painful aspects of human existence:
We become too attached to life and its benefits. We become
overly attached to our spouses, parents, children, reputation, ambitions, and ideas. Giving them up voluntarily is
painful enough, but when they're taken away, it's unbear-

able. What if we were not so attached to them? Are we afraid we might become callous, unfeeling? Yet the central call of the gospel is that we are to let go of all we cling to and find our security in an eternal savior.

Seven Steps to Healing

This is Dr. Hart talking, and out of my own counseling experience I've identified seven distinct steps that lead to resolving reactive depressions. You can try to work through these steps by yourself, but I would strongly encourage you to do so with the help of a friend or counselor. Each step will lead to the next, and along the way, it will be helpful for you to journal the process as you grow and heal.

Step 1: Identify the Loss

Some losses are easy to recognize. They are tangible, measurable, and certainly visible. Others are not. They are hard to pinpoint and grasp. They may only be ideas in your head or vague feelings. But since we can only grieve what we know to be lost, the first step in resolving a reactive depression is to identify what has been lost.

Very few losses in life are simple. Each major loss may represent many minor losses. A major loss is like a diamond with many facets or faces. It is these facets that give a diamond its brilliance. The more facets there are, the more a diamond sparkles. Losses, also, have many facets. For example, being fired from a job is not a single loss, but many. There is the loss of wages (a real loss), the loss of status that comes with being a gainfully employed person (an abstract loss), the loss of face or the feeling of humiliation at having to tell one's spouse and friends that you've been fired (also abstract). There is also a threatened loss

of not being able to get another good job, a loss of friendships in the workplace, and a loss of familiar surroundings
and pleasurable routine. And this is only the beginning;
you must unravel all of them so you can see the whole
picture.

Step 2: Understand All the Facets

The second step is to develop a more complete understanding of the full complexity of each loss. Every facet
needs to be brought into focus in such a way that it will
help your mourning. Each of us will experience the same
loss differently. We each have our distinctive emotional
fingerprints; we differ in our history of losses, in our values, and in our worldviews. Some of us might place more
emphasis on social values, others on material loss.

Step 3: Separate the Concrete from the Abstract

All losses and all aspects of a given loss can be divided
into two general categories, concrete or abstract. It helps
if you can separate the concrete aspect of your loss from
the abstract, because the concrete, or real losses, are easier to let go of.

Abstract losses are the more difficult to grasp, and consequently the more difficult to grieve. They may exist only
in the mind, but they nevertheless do exist. Loss of love,
self-control, self-respect, ambition, a sense of God's presence, self-mastery, and the respect of others are all examples of abstract notions that can be lost.

Concrete losses may be easier to overcome, but they
may have significant abstract losses attached to them.
Here's an example: Suppose I submit a manuscript to a
publisher, and it is rejected. The concrete loss (return of
the document with accompanying letter of rejection) is

the least significant loss. I can always try another publisher. The more significant loss will be the effect of the rejection on my feelings about myself. I will probably tell myself that I'm no good. I will question my competence and irrationally (I hope) think that I'll never ever again be able to write another book. I will conjure up visions of many rejections, and all the while I will be creating further losses, which will only make me more depressed.

The better I understand these losses, however, the easier I can sort out the sense from the nonsense so that I only grieve the sensible. Because abstract losses are less tangible, they lend themselves to all sorts of distortions and imaginations. You need to bring your grieving process back to the real world.

Step 4: Separate the Imagined and Threatened Losses from the Real

Besides the categories of concrete and abstract losses, there are imagined and threatened losses. These are important to identify, because the grieving process can only be completed for the real losses. In other words, you can't grieve imagined losses, nor can you complete the grieving of threatened losses.

If your loss is imagined or has imagined components, you must attempt to convert them to real losses. If you can't, discard them. You can do this by testing reality, or finding out the truth. If you are depressed because you fear you might have breast cancer, for example, go to the doctor and have it checked out. If you try to live with imagined fears, they will only make you depressed. Since there's nothing to grieve, you can't get over these imagined losses. This is how a great deal of depression is perpetuated.

Similarly, threatened losses begin the grieving process, but since no actual loss has taken place, you cannot complete your mourning.

Step 5: Facilitate the Grieving Process

One of the consequences of exploring the full implications and feelings of a loss is that it will intensify the feelings of depression. This is important because it facilitates the grieving process. It may seem paradoxical, but in reactive depression, the more deeply we experience our depression, the more quickly we recover. Fighting off the depression or trying to minimize the pain of it only serves to prolong it.

Once you feel that you really understand your loss, move to facilitating the grieving process by allowing the feelings of depression to intensify. Give yourself permission to feel the pain. Stop yourself from running away from it. Healing takes place when you allow yourself to go through the grieving process.

Give yourself permission to grieve and feel depressed, at least for a certain amount of time. Your body, mind, and soul will tell you when it's over, but if you don't start it, the grieving never finishes!

Step 6: Face Up to the Reality of the Loss

The ultimate outcome of reactive depression is to help you let go. The sooner you accept the reality of the loss—assuming that there is a real loss—the sooner you will recover from the depression.

In this step, therefore, you face up to and accept the reality of the loss. Denial is common at the start of a depression. Wishful thinking tries to restore or delay the loss. Both need to be prevented. Prayer is crucial here. God comes to us in such painful moments with comfort and reassurance.

Step 7: Develop a Perspective on the Loss

This step follows naturally from the previous one. The loss has to be placed in the context of the larger perspective on life. It is here that knowing God through Christ must make a difference in the way we adjust to loss. It gives us a vantage point from which we can evaluate our losses and interpret our future. It gives us hope that despite life's terrible blows, there is a future for us. This is essentially a spiritual step and should be facilitated through prayer and the power of God's Spirit.

A Final Note

Women can suffer from very deep emotional wounds from the losses they experience in life, wounds that cut into the depths of their very beings. When a woman becomes deeply depressed and does nothing about it, she damages not only herself, but also everyone she loves and who loves her.

The grieving process we have described in this chapter is essentially a normal process in that we all have the capacity to mourn and adjust to our losses. To be healthy, we must learn to grieve our losses. If we don't allow ourselves to grieve or get stuck in the grieving process, normal depression becomes clinical depression, and professional help becomes a must. If you feel that you have lost control of your grieving process, we strongly encourage you to get help right away. Refer to part 3 on getting the help you need.

5

Stress, Anxiety, and Depression

God, I won't fret or have anxiety about anything,
I will not let my heart be troubled or afraid.
Instead, in every circumstance, I will pray with definite
requests and thanksgiving, continuing to shape my worries into prayers.
Then I know that I will have your peace, and a tranquil
state of my soul, which will guard my heart and my
mind.

Prayer inspired by Philippians 4:6–8; John 14:27

Surprise, surprise: Prolonged, excessive stress is one of the major causes of anxiety and depression in women. Stress can also be the cause of a wide variety of physical ailments. Clearly, it's a byproduct of our advanced, technological, driven, modern-day civilization—and the current epidemic increase of stress-related illnesses and depression is unlike anything we've ever seen. All this, despite the paradoxical advances that have been made in medical science.

Somehow, we're faced with more complexity and deteriorating factors than before, and the result is that we're "overstimulating our stress-response systems . . . and many of the solutions are too complex for success-ful resolution."[1]

So How Do Women Fare?

Obviously, women have not escaped the stress of today's fast-paced world. In fact, they may feel it even more than men. Juggling professional life, career decisions, education needs, family schedules, money concerns, child rearing, and child care isn't easy for anyone. Working mothers in particular, whether married or single, are probably at the top of the list of those facing higher levels of stress, both at work and in the home.

Everything changes so fast these days, and that's just one of the factors that can increase stress for an already-burdened woman. Add to that complexity, plus a decrease in social connection and recovery time, and you'll see that in many cases, priorities are unbalanced. Women are being impacted by increased noise, polluted air, and "hurry sickness." Emotionally, women now have to worry about where the money is going to come from like never before. Personally, we don't know any women who are not frustrated and overloaded, trying to find the balance between work and family. Many feel afraid, insecure, and isolated.

But stress isn't only a physical problem. Women also struggle spiritually, and many feel "inner emptiness." They lack meaning, purpose, and hope for the future. Social connections and support systems are being severed through widespread divorce and separation, marital strain, and the unfortunate lifestyle of the busy commuter. This chronic strain and disconnectedness are contributing more significantly to stress disease and depression than most of us realize.

Stress Can Be Constructive

Before we delve any further into the relationship between stress and depression in women, it's important to note that not all stress is bad. No one can live without experiencing some degree of stress. Simply getting in the car and driving across town can be stressful—especially if you have to take a freeway. Rushing to complete dinner arrangements after a busy day at work can be stressful. Being a mother with young children at home is stressful. But so is the sheer joy of seeing your daughter win a determining soccer game. The grandfather of all stress research, Hans Selye, has said that stress is the spice of life, for any emotion, and activity, causes stress.

Some of the everyday stresses and challenges in life facing you as a woman today can actually be good for you—if you can learn to keep it under control. Stress can stimulate growth mentally, physically, or spiritually. This positive, constructive form of stress is known as "eustress," and it stretches us, gets us to reach for our goals, or motivates us to explore new options in life. It is what helps us get the house cleaned before guests arrive or what gets a mom up in the middle of the night at the cry of her baby. This constructive kind of stress can also energize us, giving us creativity before meeting an important deadline. Yes, trials, difficulties, and deadlines in life can be very stressful. But from God's perspective, these stressful times are essential for building our maturity and character.

When Is Stress Destructive?

To put it bluntly, the only good stress is short-lived stress. It's when it's prolonged that things get out of hand. Unfortunately, we've entered an era in which women are not only undergoing an enormous increase in levels of stress, but that stress is also chronic; it never goes away. And we pay the price through stress-related diseases like heart problems, panic/anxiety problems, and of course, depression. Dr. Richard Swenson, M.D., discusses the effects of

stress he has seen as a doctor in his book *Margin.* Every fifteen minutes, he wrote, people come through his office exhausted and hurting—and since the American Academy
of Family Physicians estimates that two-thirds of office visits to family doctors are prompted by stress-related symptoms, Swenson has seen a lot of stress-related damage.

It is absolutely essential, therefore, that women today
pause and reflect on how they can reduce and manage
stress, what the stressors are in their lives, what their perceptions are of those stressors, and how their stress, if it
went out of control, could harm every aspect of their lives.

So What Is "Stress," Anyway?

Ask around, and most people will tell you that stress is
a bad thing. But this is Dr. Hart here, and if there's one
thing that amazes me, it's that few people can actually
identify the really bad stress in their lives. Most people
look at the "bad" things happening to them as stressful.
Unfortunately, some good things also become stressful
when they're prolonged.

Let's pause for a moment here and define a few important concepts: stressors, stress, distress, and stress disease.
Each one leads to the next, and a greater understanding
of each will definitely be beneficial.

First comes the "stressors." A stressor is an external
demand or environmental change that triggers an increase
in our stress response, the so-called "fight or flight" mech-
anism. Stressors can come in the form of major life events
like birth, divorce, or loss, or may involve chronic strain
like relationship conflict, financial pressures, or busy
schedules. Daily or occasional strains like change, a sick
child, or a traffic jam on a Friday afternoon are also stress
contributors. Other stressors on our systems can come
from environmental toxins or physical trauma. American

adults (both men and women) usually cite finances, family, and the chronic strain of work as their top stressors.

So what are the stressors in your own life? Here's a list of things that could be bothering you.[2] Mark all those that apply, then see what you can do to improve the situation.

External or physical stressors

Death: loss of a spouse, loved one, or close friend

Marital problems: divorce, separation, conflict

Trauma or crisis

Physical illness

Disability

Conflicts with people at work or neighbors

Pregnancy: wanted or unwanted

Work/career changes: Being fired, changing to a new job/career

Balancing work and family

Relationship strain, disconnection

Financial pressures

Life changes

Barriers that prevent you from reaching your goals

Excessive or impossible demands on you at this stage of your life

Boring, lonely work or an unreasonable boss

Internal stressors

Feelings of helplessness

Irrational ideas about how things should or must be; perceiving that life is not unfolding as you think it should

Believing you are incompetent, helpless, or can't handle a situation

Catastrophizing or drawing faulty conclusions

Pushing yourself to excel and/or failing to achieve a desired goal

Blaming yourself or others for bad events

History of intense stress, especially in childhood, which can predispose you to overreact to current stress

Unexpressed feelings or internalized anger

When your boss tells you that she wants a certain project completed before you can go home, the demand is a stressor. When your kids are cooped up inside for an entire rainy day, screaming and running around the house, their behavior and the situation is a stressor. Stressors cause an increase in your emotional and physiological stress response; they are not the stress itself. If you put earplugs in your ears, you can shut out the noise that is stressful. By going to a movie, you could get the kids out of the house and quieted down. You might even be able to sit down during the movie, breathe deeply, and calm yourself, which would lower your stress response. In other words, we can always control our level of stress by controlling the impact of stressors on our lives.

Interestingly enough, the same stress that makes one person sick could be invigorating to another. Personality styles, perceptions, previous experiences, lifestyle, relationships, and the location where we live are just a few factors that impact individual differences in stress tolerance and ability to recover.

It's important, then, to learn your limits and accept them. Develop an adequate system of recovery and know when to pull back from the edge of overstress. These skills are essential to avoiding depression. Our goal here is to show you practical lifestyle strategies that can help to reduce the effects of excessive stress.

So when confronted with a major stressor, you have a few options. First, you can simply accept the situation; there may be nothing you can do to change it, but by accepting it, you can reduce its impact. Second, you can avoid the situation; this will diminish your frustration and avoid other stressors. Third, if possible, you can alter the situation; making changes, choices, or adjustments can sometimes relieve the stressors. Or last, you can adapt and change your response to the situation; even if you can't change the stressor, you can find ways to manage the stress effects, and you can change your attitude toward it.

Feeling a Little TENSE?

Now that we've looked at stressors, let's look at stress itself. Stress is physical, mental, and/or emotional strain in response to a demand, pressure, or disturbance. Physiologically, stress is the arousal of our adrenal system, which releases hormones into the blood stream to help us cope with the emergency. Just opening your eyes in the morning after a good night's rest is stressful, because it wakes up the adrenal system. The very act of living imposes a measure of stress on our body and mind. Stress, then, is a normal physiological response when it helps us respond and adapt to change. Our adrenaline surges and stress hormones are sent all over the body to prepare us for either a fight or flight. But when the adrenaline is allowed to continue rushing throughout our bodies, it begins to be destructive, resulting in burnout, exhaustion, and depression.

Ah, So Distressed!

Distress, the third part of the stress response, occurs when our stress response is intense and/or prolonged. At this point, stress symptoms start to set in; this has also been called overstress. A short period of high stress can be just as damaging as a long period of less intense stress, so both must be watched. If a headache starts within minutes of arriving home from work, your system is in distress mode. In one sense, the headache is a distress signal, telling you you've gone too far this time. Distress can, therefore, be a warning sign— if we heed those warnings.

Symptoms of Excessive Stress

Listed here are some of the possible manifestations of too much stress in your life. Indicate the ways you are experiencing stress now.

0 = Never   1 = Sometimes   2 = Often   3 = Always

Physical
__ Chronic fatigue; exhaustion
__ Sleeping problems
__ Aches and pains
__ Headaches
__ Frequent colds or flu
__ Severe loss of appetite (anorexia) or inability to stop eating
__ Stomach/digestive problems such as indigestion, constipation, loose stools
__ Listlessness
__ Dark circles under the eyes
__ Tightening of muscles in head and neck
__ Rashes; itching
__ Nervous ticks; tremors

Emotional
__ General dissatisfaction
__ Loss of enjoyment in life
__ Irritability; impatience
__ Inner turmoil
__ Depression
__ Angry outbursts and hostility
__ Moodiness
__ Stewing in anger rather than expressing it
__ Nervousness; tension
__ General feeling of being overwhelmed
__ Guilt; self sacrifice
__ Disillusionment
__ Anxiety
__ Apathy

Mental
__ Inability to concentrate
__ Forgetfulness
__ Pessimism
__ Confusion
__ Lethargy
__ Rumination
__ Churning and busy mind
__ Excessive worry
__ Mental fatigue

Social
__ Feeling lonely and unloved
__ Isolation; alienation; withdrawal
__ Lower sex drive
__ Sexual problems or concerns
__ Trouble with relationships, such as not getting along with family and friends
__ Inability to take criticism
__ Inappropriate laughing
__ Nagging/yelling at others

In addition, add point values to the following statements:

__ My stress is caused by forces beyond my control
__ I feel as if my life is spinning out of control
__ I feel pressured by my commitments
__ I feel like running away
__ I feel stuck in a rat race
__ I have trouble relaxing
__ I feel tense and rushed
__ No matter how hard I try, I never feel caught up
__ I feel burdened by financial problems
__ I have difficulty setting and reaching goals

Scoring:
60–80	High stress
40–59	Moderate stress
20–39	Mild stress
0–19	Low stress

What other ways is stress impacting your life?
Other_____

If we don't, we can pay the price in eroding the foundation of our health.

The Importance of Recovery Time

Whatever the stress, it's important to remember that our adrenal systems need time for recovery from it. If they don't get that chance, they become exhausted, and depression follows.

Distress falls into two categories: recoverable and nonrecoverable. A headache is a recoverable form of distress, because no permanent damage is being caused. Back off, rest, and slow down, and it will go away eventually. But a stomach ulcer is a different level of distress; it may be nonrecoverable. If the hole is big, there will always be a scar that is vulnerable, as permanent damage may have occurred.

Depression, too, may be recoverable distress, since it will go away when you learn from it and get it under control. Some depression, however, is nonrecoverable; it may require treatment.

As long as you can counterbalance stress with recovery time, stress can be useful to your growth. It is actually in the times of recovery that personal growth occurs. When we lift weights to build muscle, it is after the workout, when the muscle is resting, that the building happens.

When it comes to stress recovery, it can happen in two ways: actively or passively. Active recovery may include some form of physical exercise as an outlet, for example. Passive recovery, on the other hand, may be done through relaxation techniques, resting, creative artistic projects, knitting, reading, journaling, taking a hot bath, prayer, or meditating.

When Stress Becomes Disease

The final phase of stress, then, is stress disease. At this point, you have developed a nonrecoverable and debilitating condition. Chronic heart disease is definitely not a recoverable form of distress; it's a full-blown disease. You'll have to live with this kind of disease the rest of your life—and that may not be too long if it's not treated professionally and a wellness lifestyle is not implemented. There are some depressions that are also considered diseases, and you may have to live with them the rest of your life, as well. Here, too, partnering with professional treatment and implementing a wellness lifestyle will be essential.

The main point we are making here is this: If you listen to the warning signs of recoverable distress, you won't have to live with the consequences of a nonrecoverable disease.

The Negative Effects of Stress

Frankly, a complete discussion of the negative effects of stress is beyond the scope of this book. If you want to read a more complete discussion, read Dr. Hart's book, *The Hidden Link Between Adrenaline and Stress*. In summary, though, here are some of the effects of chronic stress:

1. Stress symptoms can mimic a "heart attack." Symptoms such as shortness of breath, heart palpitations, chest pain, dizziness, tingling sensations in fingers and toes, and a dreadful sense of doom could actually be signs of a stress-related panic attack or a serious anxiety disorder.
2. Chronic stress and distress disease can lead to panic and anxiety attacks.

3. Stress can make you sick. Chronic stress can reduce "killer blood cells" and white blood cells, which are important for your immune system, increasing the risk of infectious diseases, viral infections such as influenza, and bacterial infections such as tuberculosis.
4. Stress can lead to exhaustion. The strain of energy, bodily resources, and the hormones required during stress finally leads to fatigue, exhaustion, and depression. The body experiences adrenaline overload and cannot stretch any further. This leads to a collapse of the system.
5. Stress can lead to severe depression. When a woman experiences excessive stress, she is more likely to become depressed. Depression also mimics some of the symptoms of stress, including changes in appetite, sleep disturbances, and lack of concentration.
6. Stress can damage your brain. Research reveals that persistent stress can actually damage your brain cells. Short-lived "fight-or-flight" stress can be good for brain functioning. Long-lasting, inappropriate stress triggered by everyday pressures such as work frustration, traffic jams, financial worries, young children at home, and relationship problems can wear down your brain. The eventual result of lasting stress is the inability to concentrate and forgetfulness.

It's a Woman Thing

One of the main reasons women seem to suffer from depression more than men has to do with their different coping styles. Basically, men and women respond to stress differently. Men are more likely to employ action and mastery strategies, such as involving themselves in activities that both distract them from their worries and give them a sense of control. Men also tend to respond to stress with

---

Symptoms of
Addiction to Adrenaline and Adrenaline Exhaustion

Symptoms:

- Intense, short duration depression
- Can't get energy going in morning
- Overcome by fatigue when "let down"
- Strange body sensations ("parasthesias")
- High irritability
- Profound negativity and bleak outlook
- Low grade depression

"acting out" behaviors such as addictions or aggression. Women tend to respond to stress with "acting in" behaviors like ruminating and other behaviors that lead to depression, including isolation, negative thinking, eating disorders, substance abuse, and poor self-care.

When It All Piles Up: Chronic Strain and Rumination

As we've said earlier, women are more likely to ruminate and dwell on their emotions. Unfortunately, these negative thoughts in turn feed the stress, and it becomes a vicious cycle. Ruminating can actually maintain chronic stress, because it drains you of the motivation, persistence, and problem solving skills to change your situation. Becoming passive, failing to do what you can to overcome stressful situations, or not taking steps to improve your environment perpetuates the strain and creates a vulnerability to depressive symptoms. So the interaction between rumination and chronic strain makes it difficult to overcome either one. This is one reason why many therapists prescribe exercise (especially aerobic exercise) as a partial antidote for chronic stress and depression. Apart from the physical benefits, it gives women an increased sense of self-discipline, control, and mastery.

For women, therefore, it is especially important to learn how to have a greater sense of control over your circumstances (and reactions to them) and problem solve rather than ruminate. Also, change what you can in your social circumstances; it will lessen the social strain that often leads to rumination.

Studies have shown that women who have multiple roles may suffer from less depression, due to the variety of support sources, connections, and outlets for their competence. If things aren't going well in one area, they can compensate by feeling satisfied with their successes in other areas. In addition, the variety of connections and support have proven to be very important for preventing and overcoming depression.

Who You Really Are and How It Fits

Another factor that impacts stress is the overlap between a woman's personality and her sense of control. To make a point, let's look at the classic Type A and Type C personality styles. The Type A person tends to be time-oriented and can harbor a great deal of anger and hostility traits, which are linked to a number of illnesses—not the least of which is heart disease. These are the adrenaline junkies, and they tend to thrive on the stress and adrenaline rush. The downside is that they don't know their limits and can push themselves to exhaustion, increasing their risk for stress-related diseases and depression. The Type C person, on the other hand, tends to be a cancer-prone personality, and also shows correlation with rheumatoid arthritis and other illnesses. They tend to be the accommodators, always putting others' needs before their own. They often play the victim, and this, along with "accepting" tendencies, can become a self-fulfilling prophecy. The victim mentality often hinders the courage and determination it takes to overcome challenges and illnesses, manage stress, and fight against depression.

Tending and Befriending

There's a new stress paradigm for women, and it adds another dimension to the stress response.[3] A new model proposes that women respond to stressful situations by "tending," or protecting themselves and their young through nurturing behaviors. This new model fills the huge gap in the stress response literature which has been mostly focused on males.

Research conducted at McGill University on rats showed that when rat pups were removed from their nests and mothers for brief periods and then returned, the mothers immediately moved to nurture and soothe their pups by licking, grooming, and nursing them. Apparently, the mother responds this way partly due to the physiological response to stress that inhibits flight: the release of the hormone oxytocin. This hormone enhances relaxation, reduces fearfulness, and decreases the stress responses typical to the flight-or-fight response. It promotes care-giving behavior, hence the idea that women respond to stress by tending.

The other aspect of the response to stress in women is "befriending." Women under stress form alliances with a larger social group, particularly other women. Men, on the other hand, show a tendency to stick more to the fight-or-flight response. Women are much more likely than men to seek out and use social support in all types of stressful situations, including dealing with health-related concerns, relationship problems, and work-related conflicts. In other words, be willing to "tend and befriend," as it is a natural and effective way to minimize the damage of stress. It builds on the brain's attachment/care-giving system and leads to nurturing behavior.

Take a Breather: Strategies for Reducing Stress

Some stressors can't be avoided. Severe loss, a difficult work environment, or an unhappy family situation cannot just be rescheduled or avoided—at least, not without tremendous cost. Here, your only option is to manage your stress. You'll need to focus on reducing its impact. Adding nurturing, positive, relaxing recreation and enriching people and events to your life will also benefit you.

As in the treatment and recovery from depression, there is no one cure that fits all stress situations. A successful strategy for treating the stress in your life will need to be tailored to your circumstances and personality. A combination of approaches is what usually works best. You'll probably have to make some changes in your life, like changing your job if possible, or even taking a leave of absence to restore your health. Staying home with your children for a while can work wonders for your perspective on life. Maybe it will mean reevaluating how you spend your evenings and weekends, cutting back on extra activities in order to give more time to personal recovery. It might mean taking advantage of modern technology and ordering groceries over the Internet and having them delivered to your front door—even brought right into your kitchen. Above all else, good stress management definitely requires that you make more time for exercise, relaxation, enjoyable restorative recreation, and making meaningful connections with friends, family, and other enriching resources.

Your Food Does Affect Your Mood

To start, let's look at what's on your plate. Many people assume that what they eat has nothing to do with their stress. Not true! When we're overstressed, the tendency is to gravitate toward food and substances that are additional triggers and generally not calming or helpful in alleviating the physiological effects of stress. Generally, the biggest culprits that can cause or aggravate stress are alcohol, caffeine, and refined sugar.

Some foods and substances can even increase stress and anxiety. These are called pseudostressors or sympathomimetics. Potential pseudostressors are found in substances containing caffeine such as coffee, tea, colas, chocolate, cocoa, and several over-the-counter drugs like Excedrin. They're stimulants that exert what is known as the "yo-yo" effect on the body, giving a brief sense of being "up," but then leaving an even greater feeling of depleted energy afterwards.

During times of stress, the brain is rapidly depleted of serotonin, the neurochemical that regulates both mood and appetite. So when you're feeling low, you will tend to gravitate toward substances and foods that give you a quick pickup, but in actuality will bring you down. Research has shown that anxiety and depression are diminished—and often vanish altogether—when sugar and caffeine are removed from the diet.

A Healthy Stress-Buster Diet

- Eliminate or restrict intake of caffeine, alcohol, refined sugars, and processed foods —any "pick-me-up" or "put-me-down" substances.
- Eat regular, planned meals in a relaxed environment.

- Eat five to six small meals a day to keep your blood sugar stable.
- Eat more fruits and vegetables. Foods with pantothenic acid can be especially helpful as well, including whole grains, legumes, cauliflower, broccoli, salmon, liver, sweet potatoes, and tomatoes.
- Drink eight glasses of water a day.
- Take nutritional supplements, including a multivitamin with minerals, extra Vitamin C, B5, B6, zinc, and magnesium; and botanicals such as ginkgo for memory, kava for anxiety, and valerian root to help you sleep. You can learn more about these in detail in the chapter on complementary medicines.
- Check for allergies and avoid foods that give you bad reactions.

Once you have determined what the stressors are in your life that cannot be avoided, the next step is to make the adjustments necessary to reduce and manage your stress. It is also important to know how you will manage and recover from ongoing stress. The amount of restoration and recovery needed by your body, mind, emotions, and spirit will all be determined by how you spend your time and energy. Sometimes you can't wait until the stressors have passed, but you may need to learn how to relax in the midst of your turmoil. Relaxation is a powerful antidote for stress. It lowers your physiological responses to stress because it is the opposite response to the fight-or-flight response. Improving the quantity and quality of your sleep is probably the most effective way for dealing with stress that can't be avoided. And as for you Type A's, learn to break your addiction to adrenaline. Here's an overview of the path to a fully restored body and mind:

1. *Identify the stressors in your life.* What are the factors that are currently causing stress in your life? Make a list of them and identify the necessary changes you need to make to reduce the stress in your life.

2. *Know how you are responding to your stress.* Identify what patterns you use to react to stress and replace negative patterns with healthier, positive ones. You can change your response to stress. Refer to the healthy lifestyle ideas and methods for managing and reducing stress later in this section.

3. *Keep a stress log.* Become aware of the stressors and stress response in your life by writing down the stressful events and how you are responding to them. This can help you identify strategies to reduce and manage stress.

4. *Know what works best for reducing your stress.* Utilize both passive and active recovery approaches. Again, active possibilities include exercising. Passive possibilities include resting, drawing, painting, knitting, starting a new hobby, finding fun activities, talking to a friend, journaling, taking a long hot bath by candlelight, getting a massage, learning relaxation techniques, praying, listening to relaxing music, reading, or watching a funny movie. Nurture yourself in whatever way reduces stress.

5. *Calm your mind and body.* Use relaxation/breathing exercises as often as you can throughout the day; take minibreaks. Learn the art of controlling your thoughts with a positive mental attitude and develop constructive, healthy thinking patterns through relaxation, meditation, and quiet reflection time. Take all your worries and cares to God in prayer. He can calm your heart and mind as you rest confidently in him. Other ways of relaxing and calming down include aromatherapy, guided imagery, biofeedback,

massage, soothing music, an enjoyable book, and a warm bath. (Refer to the chapter on natural complementary therapies for more details on stress reduction relaxation techniques.)

6. *Express your feelings and learn to manage anger.* When you keep negative thoughts and feelings stuffed inside, it's draining emotionally, mentally, and physically. Journal or talk to someone who will listen as you constructively express your feelings. That person could be a family member, a friend, a therapist, or, of course, God. Sharing these feelings with someone else relieves the strain and also strengthens the connection with the person with whom you are sharing.

7. *Friends can be good medicine.* Make meaningful connections. Utilize your family, friends, community, church, and all possible healthy, nurturing social support systems that are available to you.

8. *Give, invest in, nurture, and contribute to others.* Become outwardly directed. Volunteer, help out at church or school, or find a family in need you can make a meal for. Be kind and thoughtful toward others and be a safe, trusting connection for them. Often when we see the pain in the lives of others, it puts our own lives in perspective.

9. *Reduce relationship conflict issues.* Learn effective communication and problem-solving skills. If necessary, become more assertive. Confess, forgive, and reconcile relationships. This may require a neutral party such as a counselor so you can see both sides of the issue.

10. *Manage your time; get more control over your life.* Use a daily calendar system to organize your days, write things down, avoid putting things off, and set priorities and limits to your involvement in activities. I heard somewhere that a good way to deal with

overstress is to make a list of all the things you have to do for that day, then cut the bottom half of the list off. Remember, a big part of stress is the perception of not having control, not being able to predict the outcome, and being pessimistic. Getting your life in order will help reduce the sense of being out of control.

11. **Simplify your life.** Set priorities, limits, and boundaries in your life. You do have control! Learn to say "no" and delegate without feeling guilty. The key to preventing stress is setting priorities. What's really important? Commit to a simpler, focused lifestyle. Set realistic expectations. Spend more time on enriching, relaxing events and exercises. As Stephen Covey puts it, "The main thing is to keep the main thing the main thing."

12. **Make space for downtime and personal recovery.** Have a quiet place you can go to in your home (and in nature) for solitude, rest, relaxation, and refreshing, renewing times. This could be a little corner in your room, living room, or in the garden, and might also include occasional special places like a retreat center or day spa. In addition, leave some room in your life for rest, relaxation, enjoyable recreation, recovery, and time for meaningful relationship connections. Take occasional minivacations for a day or long weekend and an annual lengthier vacation for rejuvenation.

13. **Laugh a little.** Do a little "internal" jogging (that's what laughing is all about) and set aside some play time. Rent a funny movie, go to the drug store and read the funny cards, or read the funnies in the newspaper. When talking with friends and family, try to laugh with them, seeing the funny side of the situations in life.

14. *Stop and smell the roses.* Slow down, enjoy the here and now in the simple things of life. This is Catherine, and as I write this, I'm under tremendous stress to meet the editing and printing deadlines for this book. During the last few weeks I have been confined to my office and computer. One of the ways I am managing my stress right now is by playing inspirational music softly in the background. I have a fragrant candle burning, a vase of beautiful flowers that I received for my birthday yesterday by the side of the computer, and I sniff them occasionally. These little things can really make a difference.

15. *Keep the Sabbath rest.* God created the necessity of a weekly break from the busyness of life and activities to meet with other believers, to worship and be renewed, to rest and relax.

16. *Have a daily quiet time.* Read the Bible, pray, journal, or meditate. Just the exercise of taking the time daily (and throughout the day) to quiet yourself, focus your thoughts and feelings, come before God, and connect with his love and spirit, can reduce stress and anxiety.

17. *Get regular exercise.* Exercise is the vital component to improving mood and being able to handle stressful situations. Physical exercise is essential to active recovery from stress on your body. Exercise alone has proven to have a significant impact on improving mood, as well as increasing resilience and recovery from stress. Women who exercise regularly are much less likely to suffer from stress-related fatigue and depression. When your heart rate goes up while exercising, you begin stress recovery. With frequent exercise, the body learns to recover. Aerobic activity like brisk walking or jogging for thirty to forty-five minutes a day, four or five times a week, and lifting weights two to three times a week, will be effective. The key is that you do something you enjoy and will keep doing consistently.

18. *Make sure you get enough sleep* (eight and a half to nine hours per night is the minimum for a healthy adult). It is essential for recovery and restoration. The more restorative REM sleep you get, the more resilient you will be.

19. *Eat a healthy diet.* Eat lots of fruits, vegetables, and lean protein. They're the best protection against and the best way to recover from the destructive free radicals that are released when stressed. In addition, reduce calories.

20. *Eliminate substances that are stress and anxiety triggers.* Eliminate or restrict caffeine, chocolate, alcohol, refined sugars, and processed foods.

21. *Take nutritional supplements.* Replenish the body and support the adrenal glands. Refer to the chapter on natural complementary therapies for more details.

22. *Get professional help if necessary.* Stress can contribute to a variety of physical and emotional illnesses which should be professionally treated. If you scored high on the stress test earlier in this chapter, or are feeling depressed or have an anxiety disorder, see your doctor for a complete physical evaluation. A mental health professional should also be consulted for short-term therapy, which could be effective in resolving stress-related emotional problems.

And one more thing: There's a fun "Stress Survival Kit" on page 110. Collect all the goodies in a clear bag and use it to remind yourself that God can help you keep it all together!

Stress Survival Kit

A **candle** to remind you that even when you are surrounded by darkness, Christ's love is a fire that never goes out!

A **match** to remind you that sleep, relaxation, and exercise "relight your flame" when you feel burned out!

A **Tootsie Roll** to remind you not to bite off more than you can chew. Set priorities, goals, and boundaries!

A **Starburst** to remind you that eating healthy complex carbohydrates with protein will give you a "burst" of energy! (Sorry, not the candy!)

A **Snickers** to remind you that laughter is good medicine! (Okay, just one piece of chocolate!)

A **teabag** to remind you to take time to slow down, rest, relax, reflect, and visit with others.

A **rubber band** to help you remember to be flexible but not stretch beyond your limits!

A **pencil** to remind you to daily list your blessings, use a prayer journal, and "pencil in" time for what really matters.

An **eraser** to remind you to keep your life clean by being honest with yourself and others, asking for forgiveness, and forgiving others.

Sand to remind you not to let the strain of little annoyances get to you. Remember: It's not the mountain ahead that wears you out but the grain of sand in your shoe.

6

Depression and the Life Cycle

Even when I am going through the deep, dark valleys, and
difficult seasons in my life, I will fear or dread no evil,
Lord, for you are with me; your rod protects me and your
staff guides me; you comfort me all the way through.

Prayer inspired by Psalm 23:4

Just as no depression is the same from one woman to the
next, depressions in the same woman during different
periods of life are unique as well. In this chapter, we'd like
to look at the stages of the life cycle for the average woman,
and what depression can mean in each.

Childhood and Teenage Years

Unfortunately, depressions are appearing at earlier and
earlier ages, and young women, teens, and children may
suffer sadness, dejection, self-pity, and an overwhelming
sense of hopelessness that can last throughout a lifetime.
While the likelihood of becoming clinically depressed does
rise with age, young people, especially teen girls, are experiencing the greatest increase in depression nationwide.

Between the ages of ten and thirteen, studies have shown the rates of major depression for boys and girls are about the same: 9 percent. But at puberty, something changes. The depression rate suddenly doubles for girls, a fact that every parent of a teenage girl needs to be aware of. Basically, the rate for boys doesn't change. Risk for depression in young women peaks between eighteen and nineteen years, when most graduate high school and start college. This is the phase of life when adolescent women are transitioning into adulthood and experience many changes and losses.

Is My Daughter Depressed?

Every parent should be aware of the signs of teenage depression. Besides the symptoms of adult depression we covered in chapter 2, there are a few additional ways children and teens might manifest:

- Frequent, vague physical complaints such as headaches, stomachaches, muscle aches, and tiredness
- Problems in school such as frequent absence and poor performance
- Threats of running away from home or school
- Outbursts of shouting, crying, anger, or hostility
- Unexplained intense irritability
- Severe anxiety, panic, or fear
- Reckless behavior
- Boredom
- Racing thoughts or agitation
- Lack of interest in hobbies or friends
- Among teens, substance or alcohol abuse
- Difficulty in relationships, social isolation, and poor communication
- Desire to harm self or others

Atypical symptoms also include:

- Increased appetite, rather than decreased
- Weight gain, rather than weight loss
- Increased sleeping, instead of insomnia
- Slowing of psychomotor movements, such as slow reactions or difficulty making conversation

The persistent presence of more than a few of these symptoms should prompt parents to discuss their daughter's problems with their doctor or a psychologist who specializes in adolescence.

Types of Child or Teenage Depression

When it comes to major depression, the symptoms are the same for people of any age—with the exception of the additional problems just mentioned. Dysthymia is another possibility for this age group. It's a less severe, yet more chronic form of depression that persists for at least one year in children or teens. It's accompanied by at least two of the symptoms of major depression, including the possibility of an irritable mood, and often precedes major depression. Treatment as early as possible may prevent the depression from becoming more severe and longstanding.

As for bipolar disorder, we'd like to point out that it can be difficult to identify in children and teens. In fact, in its blatant form, it's not usually seen in children. However, any child or teen who appears depressed and exhibits ADHD-like symptoms that are severe and who has excessive temper outbursts and mood changes should be evaluated to rule out early bipolar disorder, especially if there is a family history of this disorder in close relatives.

Checking the Risks

Children and adolescents who develop major depression may have a family history of the disorder, since a genetic factor may be involved. Often a parent who experienced depression at an early age—or a parent who is currently depressed—is associated with a depressed teenager. Other risk factors include:

- Cigarette smoking, which is sometimes a form of self-medicating a depression
- Stress
- Recent loss of a parent or loved one
- Conduct and attention disorders
- Abuse or neglect; children of abuse nearly always become depressed
- Trauma, including natural disasters

But When Do They Need Help?

Most children and teens don't recognize depression in themselves. Quite honestly, it can be confusing for those around them as well. Teen emotions usually fluctuate by the day, ranging from great highs to deep lows. Also, teens can express their depression in ways that might not be recognized, as are typical symptoms like sadness or apathy. Instead, teens can be intensely irritable, have angry outbursts at the slightest provocation, have problems at school or with friends, and be involved with drug and alcohol abuse. Parents often react only to the bad behavior and don't see the underlying emotional needs and hurts that lie behind the presenting bad behaviors. To complicate this further, these bad behaviors don't make it easy to approach the teen or open doors to allow the parent to talk about his or her deeper feelings.

As a Parent, What Can I Do?

The most important thing you can do if you suspect that your child or teenager is depressed is to get professional help. Start by going to see someone yourself, before you drag your child along, just to make sure that you are not exaggerating the problem. Thankfully, many advances have been made in treatment, and an effective plan may include a combination of short-term counseling, medication, and intervention involving the home and school environment. In other words, the family could be involved in some counseling sessions, as well as the counselor working with the teachers at school. In most cases, treatment should continue for at least six months to prevent recurrence. Refer to the chapter on getting the help you need for guidance on counseling and medication.

In the meantime, consider the following:

1. ***Create a safe place to talk.*** Children and teens need an opportunity to talk about their sadness and other feelings. Depressed children and teens are often unable or unwilling to talk directly about how they feel. They aren't able to name and identify their primary emotions, so instead they act irritable, sullen, and angry, especially towards their parents. This escalates conflict and spirals into increased isolation, feeling alone in their pain. These children and teens need to have a safe place to learn to talk about their feelings, frustrations, and challenges. This could be provided by a parent, family member, teacher, youth worker, pastor, or professional counselor.

2. ***Work at resolving underlying family conflicts or other causes of depression.*** Children and teens need help in identifying the causes of their depression and in learning healing ways to find resolve. This is usually

done under the guidance and support of a professional counselor who is experienced at working with child and teen depression and/or group counseling under the leadership of a counselor.

3. *Learn healthy relationship, emotional, and thinking skills for yourself,* so that you can model these for your children. Children and teens who are not able to resolve relationship conflicts can be vulnerable to depression. Teens are especially vulnerable to romantic relationship hurts and rejections and need guidance and skills to help them through the immediate situation, as well as to prevent future predisposition to depression.

4. *Remember: Pessimistic habits of thought can also predispose children and teens to react to life's small defeats in negative ways.* Teaching children and teens more productive ways of looking at their difficulties lowers their risk of depression. They can also learn to challenge the thinking patterns associated with depression, to make friends more easily, to get along better with their parents, and to engage in more social activities they enjoy.

5. *Always stay connected with your children.* Many studies have been done to determine risk factors for teens and depression. But at least one study looked for variables that would be most protective against depression.[1] They discovered that the first protective factor was parent-family connectedness. This was defined by feelings of closeness, being cared for, and feeling loved and wanted by family members. The other protective factor against depression was a sense of connectedness at school and with friends, feeling that people are treated fairly at school, that they are close to people and friends, and that they're part of the school. Clearly, according to the study, the feeling of being connected is essential in the fight against

depression. Do whatever you can to build resilience in your children and help them find their place.

The Female Hormones

When it comes to hormonally related depressions in women, we can't ignore the "estrogen/serotonin dance." As we've already discussed, depression in women of child-bearing age is linked to times of low estrogen levels: just before menstruation, just after the birth of a child, and finally, toward the end of childbearing ability. It appears that there is a relationship, even a dependency, between estrogen and serotonin. Whenever estrogen drops, so does the serotonin level in certain brain cells, and this creates a state of depression. Every woman—and let's include men here also—needs to be aware of this relationship. In a moment, we'll look at the three most important effects of the estrogen/serotonin dance, namely on menstruation (PMS) childbearing (postnatal depression) and menopause (menopausal depression).

Most women have problems relating to their menstrual cycles, beginning in puberty and continuing through the childbearing years. In fact, about 80 percent of women experience physical, emotional, and behavioral symptoms that range from mild to severe. Usually these symptoms appear five to ten days before a period and disappear within a day or two after a period starts. These symptoms are usually normal and do not result in disabling distress or impair daily functioning. However, between 20 to 40 percent of women experience "mild to moderate" problems, and 2 to 10 percent have symptoms severe enough to dramatically interfere with their daily life functioning, relationships, and work life. Understandably, these problems increase a woman's risk for depression.

Premenstrual Syndrome (PMS)

Premenstrual syndrome includes a range of symptoms usually felt several days to two weeks before a woman's period. The most frequently reported symptoms include: mood swings; depression; hopelessness; emotional outbursts of crying, yelling, or anger; anxiety; feeling "on edge"; fatigue; lethargy; insomnia; nervous tension; difficulty concentrating; feeling overwhelmed or out of control; swelling or bloating; breast tenderness; appetite changes; food cravings; and aches and pains. The most common symptoms reported with moderate or severe PMS are the same as those for depression, such as low mood, fatigue, appetite changes, sleep difficulties, and decreased concentration.

For women who experience depression symptoms during their monthly cycle, the boundaries aren't always clear. Studies have shown that 30 to 76 percent of women who were diagnosed with PMS have a lifetime history of depression, compared to the 25 percent of the general female population. It's also common for women experiencing depression with PMS to have a family history of depression. Women who have depressive disorders often experience more severe symptoms around their cycles.

There is a strong overlap between PMS and atypical depression, or depression that includes the classic sadness. They share many of the same symptoms, and both disorders are believed to involve the serotonin system, which affects mood and behavior.

Premenstrual Dysphoric Disorder (PMDD)

To the great relief and validation of many women, a severe form of PMS is now a legitimate and official diagnostic category in the 4th edition of the *Diagnostic and Statistical Manual of Mental Disorders (DSM-IV)*. The symptoms are essentially comparable to those of major depression, such as depressed mood, marked anxiety or tension, mood swings, irritability, and decreased interest in activities. However, they are severe before the menstrual cycle, diminish after menstruation begins, and include other criteria.

Please note that the diagnosis of PMDD does not necessarily include all women who experience severe premenstrual stress. Just as with the diagnosis of clinical depression, there are typical as well as atypical symptoms for the disorder, which cover a broader range of each woman's experience of symptoms. Don't exclude yourself if you don't find your predominant symptoms listed. Keep a record of symptoms daily and get help from a doctor who has effectively treated women with PMDD.

According to the *DSM-IV*, here's the criteria: In most menstrual cycles during the past year, five or more of the symptoms below (including at least one of the first four symptoms) must have been present during the first week before menses. Symptoms should have diminished after the onset of menses, and be absent the week following menses:

- Depressed mood, hopelessness, negative thoughts
- Anxiety, tension, being "on edge"
- Mood swings, feeling suddenly sad or tearful, sensitivity to rejection
- Irritability, persistent anger, increased interpersonal conflict
- Decreased interest in usual activities
- Difficulty concentrating
- Fatigue, lethargy, lack of energy
- Appetite changes, overeating, food cravings
- Sleep difficulties, either insomnia or hypersomnia
- Feeling overwhelmed or out of control

Physical symptoms include: breast tenderness, swelling, headaches, joint or muscle pain, bloating, and weight gain.

In addition:

- The symptoms greatly interfere with normal functioning
- The symptoms are not merely an exacerbation of another disorder
- The symptoms are confirmed by prospective daily ratings for at least two consecutive menstrual cycles

Alleviating the Symptoms of PMDD

For mild premenstrual problems, lifestyle changes in diet, exercise, and natural supplements can alleviate many symptoms. Please don't dismiss this as too simplistic. These basics are showing significant positive results for long-term relief of PMS symptoms. Women who have consistently integrated these healthy changes in their lives over the course of a few months have noticed great improvement. For moderate to severe symptoms of PMDD, you will want to consider medical treatments such as antidepressants as well. Following are some of the effective strategies and treatments you can also consider implementing.

1. Make Changes in Your Diet

- Eat six mini-meals a day and don't skip a meal. This will help maintain steady blood sugar levels, which can help prevent mood swings. You will be amazed how much this will help, especially if your eating schedule has been erratic.
- Choose good sources of protein: fish, soy products, egg whites, legumes, lean beef, skinless chicken breast, and turkey breast.

- For every meal, divide your plate into three parts: 60 percent complex carbohydrates like whole grains, fruits, and vegetables; 30 percent lean protein; and 10 percent fat, such as olive or canola oil, avocado, flaxseed oil, nuts, or seeds.

- Reduce or eliminate your intake of caffeine, sugar, salt, alcohol, refined and overly processed junk food, excessive dairy products, and high-fat and sugary foods, especially during the two weeks before your menstrual period.

2. Exercise Frequently

Exercise is a highly effective way of reducing PMS symptoms. Aerobic exercise raises the body's level of endorphins and other chemicals produced in the brain. These are natural feel-good hormones. Some experts theorize that endorphin levels drop during the premenstrual period, leading to anxiety and depression. Exercise can help bring these levels back up, and thus alleviate the uncomfortable symptoms.

3. Reduce Stress

Reducing the sources of stress in your life—as well as utilizing mind and body treatments—has proven effective in relieving PMS symptoms. The stress-reducing relaxation response is an effective treatment for physical and emotional premenstrual symptoms, and it is most effective in women with severe symptoms. Refer to the chapters on stress, anxiety, and depression (chapter 5) and natural complementary therapies (chapter 9) for strategies on stress reduction and relaxation techniques.

4. Take Natural Supplements

Although you might be eating a healthy diet, you're probably not getting all the vitamins and minerals you need to fight PMS alone. Supplements can help give your body the extra nutrients needed to keep balanced. We'll talk more about supplements in chapter 9, but here are a few to talk to your doctor about when referring to PMS symptoms in particular:

Calcium carbonate 1,000 mg daily

Vitamin B6 200 mg (take only as recommended by your doctor, as high doses are toxic)

Magnesium 400 mg

Evening Primrose Oil 1,300 mg

Kava Kava 50–150 mg, seven to ten days before your period for anxiousness

St. John's wort 600–900 mg, divided into two or three doses with meals for mild depression

5. Consider Medication

Clinical studies suggest that approximately 60 to 70 percent of women with premenstrual symptoms reported a significant improvement with selective serotonin reuptake inhibitors (SSRI) treatments such as Prozac, Paxil, Celexa, Zoloft, and the like.

For severe symptoms of PMS and PMDD:

- *Talk to a gynecologist* who is knowledgeable in treating premenstrual symptoms. Several prescription medications and supplemental hormonal therapies are available. You have to find out what is right for you. Treatment should be designed to fit your specific symptoms, physical history, and current health.
- Your doctor can advise you on the best *antidepressant medication* to deal with your drop in serotonin. There is no one-size-fits-all serotonergic antidepressant that will cover every woman's needs. Many SSRIs have been researched and found effective.

- *Estrogen-containing birth control pills* are helpful in regulating your menstrual cycle and in alleviating some severe symptoms of PMS. Again, check with your doctor to see if this is something you should consider.

- *Hormone therapy* is a treatment consideration in very severe cases, when a woman is incapacitated by depression symptoms around her cycle.

6. Schedule Your Life according to Your Monthly Cycles

Be kind to yourself. Self-care and nurture includes being aware of your cycle and symptoms and not scheduling anything really important on the days during your cycle that are typically the most difficult. There are times that this will be unavoidable, and you will have to tough it out as best you can. However, when possible, don't schedule big meetings or major events that will be too overwhelming.

Childbirth and Beyond

When it comes to having a baby, depression can be a real problem. There are two types of problems, however, that range in their severity.

1. Baby Blues

It's not uncommon to hear a woman say, "I wanted this baby so much and now that I have it, I feel so blue." In fact, about 50 percent of new moms experience the "baby blues," crying for no apparent reason, feeling sad or anxious, or having trouble sleeping. It can happen during the ten days after giving birth and is most common around the third day. The feelings are quite natural, however, and

90 percent of the time, will subside without treatment. So what causes them? Hormones, for one thing. But that's not all. According to the book *What to Expect When You're Expecting* by Arlene Eisenberg, other factors may include:

- *The shift from center stage to back stage.* The baby is now the star. You were once the pregnant princess, but now you're the postpartum Cinderella.
- *Hospitalization.* You may be frustrated not being in control, just wanting to get home.
- *Going home.* Once arriving home, you might feel overwhelmed and overworked, especially if you have other children and no help.
- *Exhaustion.* You could be very tired from a difficult labor, not getting enough sleep while in the hospital, and then having to take care of the baby on top of that.
- *A sense of disappointment in the baby.* The baby might look small, red, and puffy, and not like the picture-book baby you had imagined. Your guilt for this might also contribute to depression.
- *A sense of disappointment in the birth and/or in yourself.* If you had expectations that didn't work out the way you had planned, you may feel you've failed.
- *A feeling of anticlimax.* The whole nine-month build up and preparation is all over now, and that could feel like a letdown.
- *Feelings of inadequacy.* New mothers can feel overwhelmed with the responsibility of caring for and feeding a new baby. The reality can be much more stark than imagined.
- *A sense of mourning the old you.* If this is a first child, you will enter into a new role and, at least for a sea-

son, leave behind the flexible, free, or career-fulfilled life.

- *Unhappiness over your looks.* When you were pregnant you had an excuse to be fat. Now you're just fat, and you're reminded of that fact because you have nothing to wear that fits.
- *New family conflicts.* These could include naming the baby, grandparent stress and expectations, choosing godparents, and circumcision decisions, just to name a few.
- *And finally, how about "paternal blues"?* Let's not forget the adjustments that the father has to make with a newborn in the house. If he was really involved in the birthing process, he might also be tired and have his own emotional reactions to it all. He might also be overwhelmed if he couldn't take extra time off work.[2]

So how do you treat the baby blues? Recovery starts with lots of rest and support from your husband, family, and friends. You'll probably feel better before long. Talk to other new moms, and commiserate about your feelings and experiences. As when treating regular mild depression, do things that will help you feel nurtured and take good care of yourself. Take some time for yourself if you need it, and get as much rest as you can. Try to relax and not get stressed about everything that has to be done around the house. Most things can wait, and for now, your focus should be on resting and caring for the baby. Ask your husband to treat you to a take-out dinner and set the table up nicely with candles.

2. Postpartum Depression (PPD)

This is a little more serious than those baby blues. In about 10 to 15 percent of cases, the mild worries will develop into a severe postpartum depression, with symptoms similar to a clinical one. The connection to clinical depression at childbirth, while once quite a mystery, is clearly caused by the effect of reduced estrogen on the serotonin system.

Women who develop postpartum depression usually do so within the first six weeks, but it can appear any time up to a year after the birth. Some of these women were already depressed before or during their pregnancies or have a history of major depression. Other women at risk for PPD have a family history of depression, have a poor support system at home, or experience low self-esteem. Since those with a previous history of depression are at greater risk for a serotonin drop, they should seek treatment ahead of time to reduce the risk of PPD.

The symptoms of postpartum depression include the following:

- Excessive concern about the baby's health, becoming obsessive compulsive
- Depression symptoms such as sadness, mood changes, lack of energy, loss of interest, change in appetite, fatigue, guilt, poor concentration, or suicidal thoughts
- Feelings of guilt, loss, anger
- Irrational thinking
- Feelings of just "going through the motions"
- Excessive self-criticism of parenting skills
- Emotional detachment from the baby, even though the baby is still well cared for

The impact of PPD on a woman and her family can be detrimental, especially to the newborn infant. This is of most concern, because studies have shown how important bonding and physical and emotional stimulation are for behavioral, intellectual, and emotional growth. When a depressed mother detaches from her babies, the baby doesn't get enough stimulation necessary for growth. In these cases, the mother will need extra help in the home, as well as professional treatment.

PPD is best treated in a manner similar to the treatment of severe clinical depression. Effective integrative treatment should include a combination of counseling, support groups, antidepressant medication, and estrogen replacement medication (if needed), along with social support and healthy lifestyle changes. Treatment is essential for the baby as well as the mother.

Menopausal Depression

As for menopause, it's defined as the absence of a menstrual cycle for a period of twelve months. After that, the woman is considered postmenopausal. Most women, however, start to have symptoms leading up to menopause at about forty-six. It can begin as early as the mid-thirties, or as late as the mid-fifties.

This early phase, called perimenopause, can last anywhere from a few months to ten years. And it's during this time that a woman will experience her most challenging and painful symptoms: hot flashes, fatigue, anxiety, emotional tension, depression, mood changes, insomnia, headaches, irregular periods, loss of libido, dry skin, vaginal dryness, and a "fuzzy brain."

Estrogen levels drop significantly at this time, and this drags down serotonin levels. Once menopause is over, serotonin levels become "unlinked" to estrogen, and women are no longer at risk for this type of depression.

There is some good news here, however. Studies are beginning to show that clinical depression is not an inevitable consequence of menopause. Although about 30 percent of women do complain about not feeling like themselves or being depressed, anxious, or irritable, many others are experiencing the menopausal years as a time of transition that leads to feeling happier and more fulfilled in new and exciting ways. This is even true for their sexuality. Menopause does have its benefits.

But for those who suffer from severe depression during perimenopause, new research is continually looking for effective help. Studies are showing that hormonal changes are definitely linked to many perimenopausal symptoms, but so are other factors like an "empty nest," discomfort with growing old, mid-life reevaluation of disappointments and frustrations, and marital problems that surface after years of being distracted by a busy life and the children. Counseling in these areas of your life might help the problem. Keep in mind, too, that once again, a family history of depression increases a woman's risk.

Obviously, if your symptoms are severe, you should see your doctor or gynecologist right away. But there's growing evidence that lifestyle changes and natural resources can effectively reduce many perimenopausal symptoms with fewer side effects. Don't dismiss these somewhat basic resources as being less effective for your healing. We are now discovering, more than ever, that the most natural and safe interventions are readily available in our everyday lives. So here's a start:

1. *Make healthy lifestyle changes.* Perimenopause provides an opportunity to evaluate your health and start choosing strategies that will enrich and protect you for the next phase of your life. Consider reducing your stress (which can impact hormonal fluctuations) and learning both active and passive ways for relaxing (see chapter 5 on stress, anxiety, and depression). Be sure you get enough sleep, taking naps during the

day if you're kept up by night sweats. In addition, stick to a healthy eating plan and exercise at least four days a week with both strength training and cardiovascular exercises. As with treating depression in general, you will need the support of your close friends and family, and maybe a support group or professional counselor. All the resources available throughout this book can be applied to overcoming depression during perimenopause.

2. *Take natural supplements.* These may include: eating soy, drinking plenty of water, taking vitamin E, taking a tablespoon of flaxseed oil daily, calcium and magnesium, folic acid with vitamin B, taking evening primrose oil daily, and using a natural progesterone cream under your arms or inner thighs twice daily. Refer to chapter 9 on natural complementary therapies for additional resources.

3. *Medical interventions.* If you have been experiencing distressing and uncomfortable perimenopausal symptoms, be sure you're with an OB-GYN who is able to effectively treat you through these years and is familiar with lifestyle, nutritional, and complimentary medicine as well. This will be difficult and might mean working with two or even three doctors.

Remember, hormonal replacement therapy should only be considered in severe cases when nothing else has worked and when there is also a high risk for heart disease, osteoporosis, Alzheimer's, and maybe colon cancer.

For moderate to severe depression, an antidepressant along with counseling has proven to be an effective treatment. Otherwise, according to OB-GYN expert Dr. Joseph L. Mayo, coauthor of *The Menopause Manager*, nutritional medicine and other complementary approaches—coupled with lifestyle changes and stress reduction—can do wonders.

PART 3

Getting Help
and Healing
Depression

7

Counseling Therapy

I thank and praise you, God and father of my lord Jesus
Christ.
You are the father of sympathy, and the God who is the
source of every consolation and comfort and encouragement.
You comfort and encourage me in every trouble, calamity,
and affliction, so that I may also be able to encourage and
comfort others who are in any kind of trouble or distress,
with the same comfort and encouragement with which
you consoled, comforted, and encouraged me.

Prayer inspired by 2 Corinthians 1:3–4

If you could take just one nugget from this entire book,
our hope is that it would be this: Don't try to face depression alone. You need the support of others.

Unfortunately, many depressed women don't have the
benefit of a loving extended family, an understanding husband, or even a supportive church or pastor. And that's
when counseling can be the most helpful.

First Things First

So far, we've talked a lot about what goes on inside the
head of a depressed woman. But what about the rest of
her body? If you've noticed signs of depression in your-

self or someone else, a full and thorough physical examination should be the first priority. If your symptoms are very severe, you may want to ask your doctor for a referral to a psychiatrist. It is important that you rule out any possible underlying medical illness, such as heart disease or thyroid problems, or even hormonal imbalances because of the estrogen/serotonin dance we've already discussed. In addition, many prescriptions can cause or aggravate depression, so review with your doctor anything you might be taking for any reason, be it prescription or nonprescription.

Depending on the preliminary diagnosis by your doctor, you should then have a complete physical examination if you haven't had one in the last six months. If you've been suffering from severe stress, anxiety, or panic attacks, your doctor will need to check for heart irregularities as well. One common condition that contributes to depression and panic attacks in women is mitral valve prolapse, or MVP. This is not a serious condition, but it could explain your depression.

At this point, your doctor may refer you to a psychiatrist, especially if he or she feels you need antidepressant medication and is unable to prescribe it. Regardless, once all possible physical disorders and illnesses have been ruled out, a full psychological evaluation is the next step.

If you're already seeing a counselor who is not trained to do such an evaluation, request a referral to one who is. Also, a psychological evaluation can help define your personality and defense mechanisms, and these could influence the type of counseling or psychotherapy you should receive. Even if antidepressant medication is strongly indicated because of the nature and symptoms of your depression, having a clear understanding of your underlying personality can help the therapist direct your therapy toward a long-term solution.

Is Counseling God's Best for Me?

Once you've had your complete physical evaluation and considered whether or not you need to be on antidepressants, there's something else to ponder: the importance of competent, professional, supportive counseling as part of your plan for recovery. We realize that the prospect and process of this kind of treatment can be daunting for anyone, but seems particularly so for some Christian women.

There are several reasons for a resistance to counseling. First, your spouse or family may not support the idea. Going into therapy can be quite threatening to a husband who fears that his wife will share intimate details about their relationship. These details may even put the blame on him for her depression, or so the husband might think. Most often, however, discomfort with counseling is due to a lack of understanding about how it all works. Some may feel that it represents a sign of spiritual failure, or that it is a secular remedy for their problems. If this is the case, then seek out a Christian counselor or psychologist. Believe it or not, there are many of them out there, and Christian counseling will certainly not be a threat to your faith.

Healing through Talking and Listening

Remember: God intended for us to make meaningful connections with others. It only makes sense, then, that counseling can be part of God's provision as he works healing and recovery in our lives. A counselor is someone who is trained to help you develop a warm, honest, and meaningful connection. He or she can help you make these connections with others, and that alone is a valuable tool. The counseling relationship becomes a safe place to explore the complexities of your life, the underlying causes of your depression, and how that depression relates to and impacts your life and relationships. It provides reliable, consistent, uninterrupted time for you, and you alone, to be heard and valued. Counseling can also provide a "growing" place to help you clarify your priorities and values, set goals to change and move toward them, think through life choices, and become intentional in living them out.

Look at it this way: Counseling is a partnership, first with God, and then with your counselor. If we start with the idea that we are to "bear one another's burdens," as it says in Galatians 6:2 (NASB), it's easy to see that it's also God's intention that we get support, guidance, and intervention to resolve our conflicts, heal our hurts, and reconnect with those close to us.

The counseling room might be the only place that you, your husband, or your family can sit down together and talk constructively about problems.

The Scope of Professional Counselors

When it comes to choosing a counselor, many people don't have a clue where to start. To help demystify the process and clarify your options, we'll take a closer look at the world of counseling, so you can be sure you find the help you need.

First, it's important to note that, though the words "psychotherapist," "therapist," and "counselor" are often used interchangeably, there are some differences. These terms are not regulated from state to state, so counselors can vary in their levels and length of training and standards of practice. In addition, some "Christian" counselors may have training in theology or even additional degrees in theology besides their counseling training. This doesn't guarantee that they will integrate their

Christian faith in your counseling in a way that is meaningful to you, but you can ask about that on your first appointment.

There are a broad range of mental health professionals with training and expertise that could effectively treat depression: clinical or counseling psychologist, psychiatrist, marriage and family therapist, social worker, licensed professional counselor, pastoral counselor, lay counselor.

Generally speaking, the more serious the problem, the more likely you'll need someone with specialized or a higher level of training. A well-trained counselor knows his or her limitations and will refer someone who needs more specialized help when it is needed. If you feel that your counselor is out of his or her area of expertise, don't hesitate to seek a professional with a greater depth of training.

Know When to Say "When"

You might still be wondering how much help you need. The choice to seek out professional help is an individual one, but there are a few general guidelines to consider. For example, you probably need help if

- your symptoms have become obvious to you or someone close to you and affect your daily life and relationships in negative ways;
- you're not able to function as usual on the job or at home;
- your thoughts are very negative and pessimistic;
- you feel depleted of energy and sad;
- your mind has become preoccupied with thoughts about dying;

- you've noticed significant changes in your appetite or eating habits, either eating too much or too little;
- you've noticed that your sexual desire is seriously disrupted; or
- you feel so desperate that you don't know whether you can continue with life.

Remember: It's important to seek help long before symptoms get serious. The longer you wait, the more severe the depression will become and the longer it may take for recovery.[1] Refer again to Chapter 2 for more specifics on the symptoms of depression.

What's Good for the Goose . . .

Just as you are unique in every area of your life, your treatment and recovery time will be as well. Underlying causes of the depression and the length of time it's been going on make a difference, as do your response to medications and your ability to take care of yourself. Some women are self-starters, and once they're given direction, they're able to take responsibility for their healing and run with it. Others, though, need a lot of support and guidance along the way.

If your depression has a physical cause, then symptoms should diminish as the medical condition is treated. Even here, however, counseling may help you heal, as well as circumvent problems caused by the impact of the depression on your life. In reactive depressions, or those that come as reactions to losses in life, your healing will require a much more complex and intentional process of discovery that can facilitate the grieving process. You will also have to learn new strategies for dealing with stress, accepting your loss, and going through the grieving process.

Along the way, keep in mind that a "whole person" approach is clearly the best plan of action. We encourage you to think not only in terms of one treatment, but to focus on healing your "whole person." That means taking personal responsibility for your self-care and nurturing, developing freedom to feel and express your emotions, learning to dispute your negative thinking and become more optimistic, and making sure you eat well, sleep enough, and exercise regularly. Redeem your pain by using the hardship as an opportunity for growth, learning new skills and habits, developing meaningful relationships, and, if necessary, considering some natural, complementary forms of treatment to your antidepressant therapy.

Overall, the research has been clear on this fact: In treating severe depression, a combined treatment of both counseling and medication will yield the highest rates of recovery. Either counseling or medication on its own is not as effective as the two combined. It'd be nice to think a "magic pill" could cure depression on its own, but it's just not so. If your doctor recommends antidepressant therapy, make sure you get into counseling, as well.

You've Got to Have a Goal

Before you select a therapist, be as clear as possible about what sort of help you want. The most widely researched forms of therapy for depression are cognitive and interpersonal therapies. If you suffered from early sexual abuse, for example, you may need to consider one of the "depth" therapies, rather than, say, cognitive therapy.

At the outset, however, ask yourself some basic questions: What is wrong and what would I like to change in my life? What do I need to accept? What are my longings, needs, cares, hopes, and concerns? Am I constantly disappointed by unrealistic expectations? Where are my expectations unrealistic? Am I ruminating, and is my thinking negative and pessimistic? Am I under chronic strain and stress, feeling my life is burned out or out of control? What is causing me difficulty, sadness, frustration? What feelings, thoughts, and behavior patterns get in my way? How are the relationships and connections in my life? How can a therapist support and help me through this difficult time?

Pray and ask God to reveal to you the areas in your life that are sources of pain or conflict, your triggers for depression, and the areas where you can grow and find healing. Consider every area of your life, including your roles in your personal life, your immediate and extended family, your church community, your vocation, and the extended community.

The Right Fit

When looking for a counselor or therapist, don't be too hasty. When looking for a physician, you can often get a second opinion and compare diagnostic tests to decide where you should place your trust. But it's a lot easier to change a physician than a psychotherapist or counselor. Since the effectiveness of your counselor may not become obvious for many months (counseling is a slow process), you could be locked into a therapist that may not know what he or she is doing. If you can, get the names of a few therapists and request an initial meeting with each one. That way, you can determine which therapist meets your needs. The following questions and answers are adapted from an earlier book by Dr. Hart.[2]

How Do I Find a Therapist?

The best way to find a referral is by word of mouth. Talk with your friends. Find out if any of your friends know a good therapist who deals with depression, or if they know anyone who knows a therapist. If a friend or someone they know had a good experience with another kind of therapist, such as a marriage and family therapist, call that therapist. Tell the therapist that you are looking for someone in the area who deals with depression and ask if he or she could recommend one.

Next, call a reputable Christian referral source, such as Focus on the Family or the American Association of Christian Counseling(AACC). (See the appendix for contact information.) These referral sources have done the screening for you, and from there, you can call the therapists directly, talk with them over the phone, and have an initial interview. If the therapists you speak with don't work with depression, ask them who they would recommend.

If you need to find a therapist who is covered by your insurance, obtain the names of the eligible therapists in your area and ask your primary physician if he or she has any recommendations. You could also ask your pastor for a recommendation.

Does It Make a Difference If the Therapist Is a Man or a Woman?

Male therapists can work effectively with female clients, but you might not be comfortable with a male therapist at this time. If you feel uncomfortable after that first visit, consider referrals for a female therapist. Some women feel uncomfortable with a female therapist. Choose whatever gender you feel most comfortable with initially.

How Important Is the Personal Connection between Me and the Therapist?

This is very significant in choosing a therapist. Studies show that the relationship you have with your therapist is more important than the specific type of therapy they use. You must be able to experience a meaningful connection. Your relationship with your therapist will become a haven of safety in which you will learn, grow, discover yourself, and develop new and more effective ways of living intentionally. You will be spending a lot of time with this person, so make sure you like him or her, that you feel comfortable and at ease, and have no reservations.

Choose someone you believe shows insight and exhibits empathy and patience towards you, one you can be honest and open with. You will have to bond with and trust this person, so if you don't feel comfortable initially, get a consultation with someone else.

Is It Okay to Ask Therapists If They're Christians?

Don't hesitate to ask about the therapist's faith affiliation. Generally, we encourage clients to seek out a competent Christian counselor, one who integrates his or her faith in counseling in a way that is meaningful to you. If you are limited to insurance referrals, ask them if they can refer you to a Christian therapist within the group options. If there isn't one, it is still important that you get treatment for your depression, so remember that competence in treating depression is very important.

What about the Therapist's Personal Qualifications?

There are three subjective aspects to determining your compatibility with a potential therapist:

- Consider the personal aspect of the therapist. In general, what is the person's age and gender? What about cultural background and number of years in practice, and how comfortable are you with all of these? If the therapist's nonprofessional life appears to be in shambles, go somewhere else.
- Consider the therapist's interpersonal style and basic personality. Is the therapist active, passive, extroverted, introverted, cold, reserved, warm, or demonstrative? Which of these are you most comfortable with?
- Does the therapist seem to genuinely care about you and your situation? This is often a sign that he or she has the healing gifts necessary to do good therapy with you. Look for a therapist that you can connect with and feel good about. Someone else could have had a great experience with this person, but you may not connect in the same way.

What Do I Need to Know about the Therapist's Therapeutic Orientation?

A competent, experienced therapist will use a combination of approaches to meet your growth and healing needs. The preferred orientations for the treatment of depression will help you identify sources of stress and depression, help you evaluate your life choices, and examine the ways you view yourself, your relationships, and your future.

Newer brief therapies have also been found to be effective in treating depression. These approaches are problem-focused, involving you as a partner in your recovery, assigning homework, and helping you build supportive connections.

What Do I Need to Know about the Therapist's Professional Training?

Not all therapists are experienced in treating depression, and many have not collaborated with psychiatrists. In other words, they may know little about medication. In addition, there is a high degree of specialization among psychotherapists. Some only treat children, some only family and marriages. Some specialize in personality disorders or brain disorders, and so on. Be sure your therapist makes a clear statement about his or her competence to treat depression.

Picking up the Phone

Now that you know the process for choosing a therapist, it's time to get on the phone. Call each therapist you have a referral for. Most likely, you'll have to leave a message or talk to a receptionist. Then, either the therapist or an intake worker will return your call. You will be asked to complete an intake form, either over the phone or in person, before you can interview a therapist. That's a good time to ask a few important questions, such as:

- What is the therapist's experience in working with depression?
- What is the fee? How is the fee determined? Are you able to take my insurance? Are you on my HMO?
- What hours is the therapist available?
- If there is more than one therapist at the clinic or practice, how much choice do I have in which one I see?
- What kind of training does the therapist have?

- If the therapist is still in training, what kind of supervision is he or she getting?
- How long has the therapist been in practice?
- What kind of license does the therapist have?
- What is the therapist's theoretical orientation and specialty area?

Once all questions have been answered and you feel comfortable with the conversation, make an appointment for an initial consultation. Don't commit yourself to anything until after that consultation has taken place.

The First Visit

The first visit is critical in determining whether this is a good fit for both of you. At that time, the therapist will want to know what brought you into therapy and what your goals and expectations are. Try to be as open as you can. The primary goal of the first session is not to solve your problem, but to establish rapport, and rapport goes both ways. You should, therefore, feel free to set the pace of the first session.

During the session and as you leave, ask yourself: Do I feel respected? Does the therapist seem comfortable with me, and am I comfortable with the therapist? Is the therapist flexible and open to my input, treating me as an equal?

Before you go, it may be important to bring up the issue of fees again. Ask how the billing system works, and how payments need to be made. Find out if there's a policy for late payments, and what happens when appointments are cancelled or missed. Discover, too, whether insurance will cover part of your therapy, and if the therapist is a provider in your plan.

And then, after it's all over, go home and pray. Remember: There's no need to rush into anything. Be persistent and patient while looking for the right therapist, and look for a feeling of confidence that will allow you to be open and honest about your deepest feelings.

Apples and Oranges: Different Types of Therapy for Treating Depression

By now, you know that there are many forms of psychotherapy, and unfortunately we cannot describe all of them here. Fortunately, most competent and experienced therapists use a combination of various approaches and select the approach that best fits your situation. This is referred to as the "eclectic" approach.

Each approach has its strengths and weaknesses, and a well-trained therapist is aware of these. All therapy can be confusing at first, but when it comes to treating depression, you can narrow the field quite a bit. Some have the advantage of being short-term, lasting for, say, a few months, while others require a longer commitment, sometimes several years. Obviously, deep-seated problems require longer-term therapy.

That said, according to the American Psychological Association, the most effective therapeutic treatment components for supporting antidepressant medications is action-oriented, problem-solving, goal-oriented, short-term, talk therapies. Therapy should be focused and concrete, with the goal of helping you deal with the specific issues and causes related to the depression. For long-standing and deeply emotionally traumatic causes of depression, a more in-depth, long-term approach such as psychodynamic therapy will be more helpful.

The success rate in treating even the most severe depression can rise to 80 to 90 percent with effective psychotherapy that includes strategic action plans such as journaling, expressive art therapy, and homework assignments in which you are actively involved in taking action to practice what you learn. This proactive approach encourages a partnership between the doctor, therapist, and client, providing a supportive environment for growth and change. Here, then, is a closer look.

Cognitive Therapy (CT)

This approach helps a depressed woman recognize, identify, and change negative, distorted thinking patterns that contribute to depression. The focus of treatment is to change these negative perceptions and develop positive life goals, more positive thought patterns, and more positive actions and behaviors.

Interpersonal Therapy

This form of therapy was developed during the 1980s and arises from the idea that four interpersonal problem areas may lead to depression. These include: interpersonal loss, interpersonal role dispute, interpersonal role transition, and interpersonal deficits.[3] This type of therapy helps women reconnect, resolve, improve, and set realistic expectations for the relationships in their lives.

Psychodynamic Therapy

The primary emphasis here is on working through unresolved internal and external conflicts and hurts from childhood. This is a helpful focus for the many women who experience long-term depression due to having experienced early loss of a parent, childhood trauma, and/or abuse. The counseling relationship explores these early experiences and repressed feelings, and provides insight to current problems and how they can be changed. The length of this approach could be as brief as a few months or continue for several years.

Supportive Psychotherapy

Here the focus is to offer you support and help during difficult times of stress, change, loss, and illness. The therapist comes alongside you to listen, show empathy, give guidance and comfort. This might also include practical education, reassurance, reinforcement, setting limits, teaching you necessary social skills, and even referrals for antidepressant medication.

Couples Therapy

Rebuilding the marriage and reconnecting takes time, honesty, persistence, patience, and realistic expectations. The benefits of couples therapy can help both partners understand the impact of depression in their relationship and get the needed support to restore intimacy and connection. Therapy can help a couple find new ways of relating to each other that may help relieve some of the symptoms of depression. Couples therapy can also help strengthen the supportive connection for both the husband and the wife and increase the experience of intimacy in the marriage.

Family Therapy

Family therapy should be considered when the family relationships and dynamics are directly being affected by the depression. This supportive environment might be just what the family needs to understand the impact of the depression on their relationships and to find new ways of relating and connecting.

Support Groups

Support groups are a wonderful way to avoid isolation, be comforted, be empowered, and get the social support you need. Many studies have reported the value and effectiveness in recovery of support groups in treating a variety of challenges besides depression, such as cancer, infertility, AIDS, pregnancy loss, violence, and even weight loss. You can contribute to the lives of others, as well as get the benefits of encouragement, a perspective on your problems, and all the benefits of reducing stress that come with being in relationship.

How Long Will It Take?

Again, it's hard to tell how long therapy will take. It depends on many issues, including the severity, duration, and underlying causes of the depression you're experiencing. Antidepressant medications, by their very nature, may take up to six or eight weeks to take effect. The medication must be built up to its therapeutic level to avoid side effects; since antidepressants are not mind-altering drugs, there is no immediate effect. It's only after they're able to communicate their message within brain cells and the number of receptors has increased that the therapeutic effect takes place. This is also true for natural complementary options such as St. John's wort and SAM-e.

If your depression is the result of a reaction to some loss or a recent event, a different healing process will occur than if it is due to a longstanding struggle such as difficulties that arose in childhood but still negatively impact your life. Likewise, if your depression is connected to a physiological disorder, then you will need to be in treatment for that, as well. Brief therapy will help you get through any immediate difficult situations, but deeper healing, because of its multilayered, interrelated issues, takes time. Even after the immediate symptoms of depression have lifted, you may choose to stay in therapy for continued growth and healing.

When should you quit? This decision is best made with input from your therapist. Don't just stop going because you don't feel like it anymore, or you feel like you've had enough. Your therapist might suggest that you seem to be doing well enough to end the present phase of therapy, or you might tell the therapist that you feel you want to bring closure to the therapy, as your goals have been met. The therapeutic relationship has hopefully been a helpful and meaningful connection. It is both helpful to you and your therapist to have a specific time of reflection about your time together, as well as have closure to your relationship.

Get the Help You Need

Hopefully, this chapter has provided insight about just how important it is to consider therapy for treating your depression, as well as antidepressant medication where appropriate. Depression is so disruptive to your enjoyment of life, social connections, and family relationships, that for the benefit of yourself and those you love, you should consider getting help. All the forms of therapy we have presented have been shown to be surprisingly effective in helping those who are depressed. After therapy, clients not only report a reduction in their depressive symptoms, but also improvement in their social and family interactions. In addition, their spiritual life is also restored. You, too, can once again resume a rich and meaningful relationship with God, and this is probably the most important reason of all for getting the help you need.

8

Antidepressant Medication Therapy

Thank you, God, for the hope and promise of my healing.
I know that you desire that I am well in my body, mind,
and emotions.

Prayer inspired by Jeremiah 30:17

There is so much misunderstanding—and even fear—surrounding the use of antidepressant medications that a little explanation is in order. Through this chapter, we hope to demystify the process and show that the use of medicine to treat depression is not only straightforward and scientific, but can also be consistent with cherished biblical principles.

Frankly, the resistance toward appropriate use of these medications is unjustified, and by perpetuating irrational beliefs about antidepressants, we cause unnecessary pain and hardship to those who are depressed.

For women in particular, knowing the connection between reproductive hormones and depression—and how antidepressants can help—is essential.

Am I Going to Get "Hooked"?

Perhaps the biggest fear people have when it comes to antidepressant medications is that they'll become addicted. So, let's put that fear to rest right at the beginning. Antidepressant medications are not addictive. You can only believe they are if you don't understand how they work. The fear of addiction is justified, perhaps, when it comes to using tranquilizers, but antidepressant medications are neither mind-altering nor tranquilizing, and they are incapable of creating an addiction. Sure, your brain will need them in order to function properly, but that's not what is meant by addiction.

Antidepressants work by helping the brain to do what it was designed to do. If nothing is wrong with your brain's neurochemistry, the medication will do nothing—unlike a tranquilizer or mind-altering drug. Don't misunderstand what we're saying here; tranquilizers may be used to treat anxiety disorders. But even here, the risk of addiction is only when the tranquilizers are abused. If your brain is deficient in its "natural" tranquilizers, the risk of addiction diminishes. If you take them when your brain is not deficient, then you are overloading your brain with tranquilizers, and addiction is a possibility.

None of this, however, applies to antidepressants. They don't alter anything in the brain directly, only indirectly—which is why they're such amazing medications. Unlike tranquilizers, which can start to alter the brain within minutes, antidepressants don't do anything right away. In fact, antidepressants can take so long to work that it can be a challenge to keep taking the medication, especially if it takes weeks to see a change. In addition, if you stop taking the medication, it may be weeks before the depression returns.

Psychological Versus Biological

If you remember from previous chapters, we discussed the difference between depressions with psychological causes and those with biological causes. Now, if we rule out obvious medical conditions that can cause depression, problems like low thyroid or severe infection, all "real" depressions are either endogenous (from within) or exogenous (from without).

It only makes sense, then, that endogenous depressions can be helped directly by antidepressants, but exogenous, or "reactive," depressions can't. Since there's nothing really wrong with the brain's chemistry in the latter type, an antidepressant may be prescribed more for its side effects than anything else. For instance, bereavement is a major "reactive" depression. If the person cannot sleep, which is quite common in bereavement, an antidepressant may be prescribed as a sedative.

So, while all depressions will include some bodily change, what we really need to discover is whether the depression is from within or without—and whether an antidepressant can help.

So How Do They Work?

The first antidepressants were called tricyclics (TCAs), but they were designed for treating schizophrenia. It was quite by accident that doctors discovered they could help treat depression as well. Later, a medication first used to treat tuberculosis was also found to help depression, and an animal tranquilizer called lithium was found to help mania.

We've come a long way since the accidental discovery method of the early days. Today, medications are computer-designed to fit certain "receptors" as they're discovered. And in just a few more years, some of the most effective antidepressants ever discovered will reach the public.

As previously mentioned, antidepressants work by inducing the brain to do what it normally does, only a bit more efficiently. They help by increasing at least two important chemical messengers in the brain, neurotransmitters, which have become depleted. These messengers are norepinephrine, abbreviated NE, and serotonin, abbreviated 5HT.

Throughout this book, we've made reference to serotonin, and knowledge about its implication in depression is rapidly becoming commonplace. It was made famous with the discovery of Prozac, perhaps the most revolutionary of all the antidepressants currently available.

Remember, though: No one medication is perfect, and it's very important to choose and monitor therapy carefully. Your biggest struggle will be to find the right medication that relieves your depression, but has the fewest unpleasant side effects. And here, everyone is different. What works for one may not work for another. Like it or not, your doctor will have to experiment with you to find the right medication or combination of medications—so be patient and cooperate.

Classes of Antidepressants

If you're going to take a medication, you might as well know how it works and what the potential side effects are. Different antidepressants target different neurotransmitters in the brain. For this reason, your doctor may suggest a change from one type to another. In the not-too-distant future, we hope to have a more scientific way of determining what particular medication a depressed woman needs. In the meantime, however, the process is still one of trial and error. So here's some background for each in the order the antidepressants were discovered.

1. Tricyclic antidepressants (TCAs): These made their mark as the first antidepressants in the early 1960s. They include elavil, imipramine, trazadone, doxepin, nortriptyline, and others. Most work mainly on one brain neurotransmitter called norepinephrine (NE), but some also work on serotonin, the other major neurotransmitter implicated in depression. They are all now available in generic form, so this means they are cheap. Unfortunately, they have a lot of side effects including sedation, dry mouth, and urinary retention. They're usually reserved for use as a last resort, but some men do better on these than on the newer ones. The TCAs do have one advantage: They help you sleep better.

2. MAO inhibitors (MAOIs): These include Parnate and Nardil, and many people who don't respond to TCAs have better luck with them. MAOIs slow down the brain's garbage collection system, thus increasing the essential neurotransmitters. The downside is that they have dietary restrictions (no aged cheese, beer, caviar, anchovies, smoked meats, or yeast products) but with the level of health consciousness we have today, there aren't usually too many complaints. There are some depressions that respond only to MAOIs. While they were always reserved for last in the "old days," today we can usually tell when they should be the first line of attack.

3. Selective serotonin reuptake inhibitors (SSRIs): This category includes Prozac, Zoloft, Paxil, Luvox, Effexor, and Celexa. The discovery of Prozac revolutionized our treatment of depression—especially in women—and opened up a whole new battery of medications that work mainly on serotonin. Despite early attacks on these medications by people opposed to all medications, they are really miracle drugs. I call them "a gift from God"—and they certainly are to those who have once again found life. These are now first-choice drugs, since they treat most depressions well and have fewer side effects than TCAs. We have yet to determine which are best suited to male depression, but we're working on it.

4. *Other antidepressants:* Several newer medications that work on combinations of neurotransmitters or have fewer side effects have now emerged, and many more are in development that could revolutionize the field of antidepressants. Truly, we are on the verge of a major breakthrough. One is called an "atypical" antidepressant, Wellbutrin, and it is used for a particular type of depression. For several of my male patients this has been the only medication to work for them. Another new medication is called Remeron, and it is selective for certain serotonin receptors, and therefore has fewer side effects.

Combine Counseling with Antidepressants

Take care when mixing antidepressants with weight reduction pills, smoking cessation aids like Zyban (buproprion), tryptophan, St. John's wort, or other substances marketed in health food stores.

At this time, there is no one best agent for the management of all depressions. Since depression in women is highly correlated with low serotonin levels (we discussed the estrogen/serotonin dance earlier) there is likely to be a strong link to serotonin-based depressions in women. This probably accounts for the huge success of Prozac with women. It works well in regular depressions, but especially well in estrogen-deficient depressions such as PMS, postpartum, and menopausal depressions.

Can one suffer from more than one form of depression? Very much so. In fact, there is hardly a biological depression that doesn't also trigger a loss of some sort due to the incapacitation it causes. So a reactive depression may very well be superimposed on a clinical or biological depression. This is probably why some form of psychotherapy or counseling, when combined with medications, shows the highest rate of success in treating depression. Using only one or the other may treat just half of the total disorder.

Coping with Side Effects

The greatest challenge you will face in getting treatment for your depression will be the management of the medication's side effects. The reason many people don't follow through on taking their medication is that they don't like the way it makes them feel. This is unfortunate, because with a little bit of experimenting, you can minimize side effects by adjusting the dose or switching to another medication. Furthermore, even problems like a dry mouth, which is the most common, lessen with time. The dry mouth problem is, therefore, easily taken care of—just carry a bottle of water with you everywhere you go. Besides, it's good for you!

What side effects should you be aware of? We've included a list of the most common. In addition to these, a woman could also experience sexual side effects such as lowered sexual desire.

What we're saying is that you'll have to put up with some side effects if you want to get better. That said, there are a few things you can do to minimize side effects:

1. Make sure you discuss your medication choices with your doctor, and weigh the pros and cons of each. For instance, Prozac may, at a high dose, cause you to have sexual difficulties, such as difficulty achieving an orgasm. Switching to Celexa can minimize this. Or, lowering the dose of Prozac and adding an

Common Antidepressant Side Effects

0 means no effect
* means mild effect
** means low effect
*** means high effect

Type	Drug	Dry Mouth	Constipation	Sedation	Insomnia	Weight gain	Dizziness
TCAs	Anafranil	**	**	*	0	*	*
	Aventyl	**	**	**	0	*	*
	Desyrel	0	0	*	0	0	**
	Elavil	***	***	***	0	**	**
	Norpramine	*	*	0	0	*	**
	Pamelor	*	*	*	0	*	*
	Sinequan	**	**	**	0	**	**
	Surmontil	**	**	**	0	**	**
	Tofranil	**	**	*	0	**	**
	Vivactil	***	***	0	0	0	*
SSRIs	Celexa	0	0	0	**	0	0
	Luvox	0	0	0	**	0	0
	Paxil	0	0	0	**	0	0
	Prozac	0	0	0	**	*	0
	Zoloft	0	0	0	**	0	0
MAOIs	Nardil	*	*	*	*	***	***
	Parnate	0	0	0	**	0	***
OTHER	Effexor	0	0	0	**	0	0
	Remeron	0	0	0	0	*	0
	Serzone	0	0	0	**	0	0
	Wellbutrin	0	0	0	**	0	0

augmentor such as lithium can stop the problem, but give you the same therapeutic effects.

2. Start your medication at a low dose and move up slowly, waiting several days between each increase. Your doctor can advise you here. If you've started high and find that the side effects are unpleasant, don't stop; merely lower the frequency with which you take the medication. For instance, ask your doctor if you can take the medication every second day

for a while, then go up. Your body will adjust if you force it to.

3. Grin and bear it for a while. Wait and see if the benefits of relieving your depressive symptoms are worth working around a few side effects.

The Good, the Bad, and the Ugly

Understanding the distinction between response and remission is essential to treatment outcome. The news is very good when you hope for a good response to treatment. You will feel better—no doubt about it. Virtually every known antidepressant has a similar response rate, about 67 percent. When coupled with psychotherapy, this response rate jumps to 85 to 90 percent. So, if you work closely with a knowledgeable physician or psychiatrist, you have a good chance of a full recovery.

So what's the bad news? Remission. Whereas we can confidently predict an improvement in up to 90 percent of depressed people who follow their treatment plan, only about 50 percent will go on to complete remission within six months. After two years, that rate goes to 67 percent. This means that quite a few women will still experience some degree of discomfort, even though they're free of the main depression.

There's one very important reason for this: depression sufferers don't pay attention to the larger "wellness" aspects of their lives. Complete and permanent recovery, a full remission, will only occur if you also change your lifestyle, lower your stress, and eat and sleep better. Attention to every aspect of your life is the only way you can achieve a complete recovery.

The best news of all is that antidepressants can reduce relapse rates after initial improvement. In other words, if you continue to take the medication after the initial six months when an improvement has taken place, your chances of relapsing into depression are less than 10 percent. Don't be too eager, then, to come off your medication; if you do, there's a 50 percent chance that you'll relapse and fall back into your depression during the next six months.

Frequently Asked Questions

Still have more questions than answers? This might help.

1. How effective are antidepressant medications?

As already shown, it is better to think about getting a good response than hoping for a complete remission. About 90 percent of endogenously depressed people can look forward to relief from depression with the right medication or a combination of medications and good counseling. You may need to be patient while various combinations are tried.

2. How soon can I expect an improvement in my mood?

Generally speaking, most antidepressants take a minimum of two weeks to take effect after you have reached a therapeutic dose in your blood stream. Several factors can slow this down. Usually you'll start at a low dose, so you'll have a chance to adjust to any side effects. Then it may be necessary to have the level of the medication in your blood checked to ensure that absorption is normal and that your liver is working properly. While taking antidepressants, avoid all alcohol, and if you have a history of alcohol abuse, tell your doctor. It could affect your response. Some antidepressants, like Prozac, could take many weeks, or even months, to make the changes that reverse the depression.

3. How long should I stay on my medication?

If this is your first episode with depression, you should probably stay on the medication for at least a year, or until your doctor advises you to stop. You should never stop on your own. If you're severely depressed or elderly, you may require a longer period of treatment. And if you suffer another episode, you may be on the medication for the rest of your life. Remember that depression is a chronic, lifetime disorder and doesn't get cured overnight.

4. What should I do if the medication doesn't work?

Ask your doctor to check your blood level regarding the medication, adjust the dose upwards if necessary, change the medication, or combine it with another. What is most important is your compliance. The problem is that these medications all take time to work, which is why they're not addicting. They give you no immediate good feelings. Consequently, when you skip taking your medication, you may still feel fine. You may even believe that, because you stopped for a few days and still feel good, you're over the depression. Not true. Remember: The antidepressant doesn't remove the underlying depression; it only suppresses the effect that causes it. If you stop taking the medication before the underlying depression is over, it returns in several weeks. Generally, the depression takes as long to return as it took to go away. In other words, try not to skip any days in taking the medication, because slowly the level in your blood will drop. If you have skipped a few days, just resume your normal dosing.

5. I've heard that some antidepressants "poop out." Is this true, and if so, what does it mean?

While the newer type of SSRI antidepressants like Prozac are quite effective, they do tend to "poop out" in about 20 percent of those who are good responders. Once you have remitted, however, you're usually beyond the pooping out risk. For a period of time, the medication may work, but then it stops working for some unknown reason, and the depression returns. At that point, your doctor may put you on another antidepressant or give you a "medicine holiday" to allow your system to become responsive again.

6. Is there any sort of test that can predict successful treatment?

Since antidepressants don't help everyone, researchers have long searched for either a subtype of depression that responds to antidepressants or a test that could predict such a response. Through the 1970s and 1980s, the search was on for a "biological marker" that could predict a positive response. The results have been disappointing, as no such test has been found that can reliably predict a good response. That could be because many types of depression are responsive to medications.

7. What if I don't have a good response to treatment?

Sometimes only some of the symptoms get better. For instance, a sad mood might go away, but motivation or an ability to enjoy things might not return. In that case, you may need to consider using multiple antidepressants. Sometimes, the depression lifts, but anxiety remains high or gets higher. In this case, your doctor may want to add an antianxiety agent.

8. What if I show no improvement on antidepressant medication?

Such depressions are called "treatment-refractory." So what are your options here? The first is to consider electro-shock therapy. This is Dr. Hart here, and I hasten to add that these days, this is not a bad option. I have recommended it, quite successfully, to a number of clients. Its bad reputation is not justified, and it will only take talking to patients who have experienced it for you to feel differently. Great care will be taken in screening you for complicating medical conditions, and the way a seizure is induced (usually restricted to one side) and the minimal amount of observable movements due to the relaxants used, make it painless and perfectly safe. The most troubling side effect is the temporary and minor loss of some short-term memory in some cases, and this is a small enough inconvenience given the potential for recovery from depression.

The Bottom Line of Not Seeking Treatment

Okay, so what happens if you don't receive treatment? There could be a high financial cost, as well as personal and social. Families are disrupted, even destroyed. Loved ones are abused, and life is wasted. Those who remain depressed for a long time lose their families or their jobs, become ill, fail to advance in school or careers, become less productive, and often turn to some form of substance abuse to relieve their emotional pain.

The most serious cost is related to suicide, the seventh leading cause of death in the United States. One out of seven people with recurring depressions commits suicide, and this makes a family's pain even more devastating. Women attempt suicide more often than men, though they are far less successful. To all Christian women who are depressed, therefore, we would say that you owe it to yourself and your family to take care of your own mental health. There is no greater gift of love a wife or mother can give.

> Taking medication seems like the wisest, sanest choice to me. Medication has not solved all my problems, but it has restored my brain chemistry to a place where I can successfully deal with the ups and downs of life. I now have stamina to go to therapy, find various resources for self nurture, and make positive decisions for myself.
>
> Carmen Renee Berry

9

Natural Complementary Therapy

Thank you, God, for creating food to nourish and restore my body, and the herbs, leaves, and other vegetation for my healing.

Prayer inspired by Ezekiel 47:12; Revelation 22:2; Psalm 104:14

I will fill my mind by meditating on what is true, noble, reputable, authentic, and kind, and on whatever is worthy of praise. As a result, I will experience your peace.

Prayer inspired by Psalm 138:7

Lately, alternative approaches to treating depression are everywhere. The Internet, the media, magazines, and self-help books are all part of the fray, touting a wide range of remedies, reporting research, and making fantastic claims. We thought it was time to clear the air.

It's true: There are many unjustifiable claims out there about remedies that are the equivalent of the old-fashioned snake oil. But there are also some very legitimate, cutting edge, and well-researched options that are worth considering. As professionals ourselves, we've tried to sort through the maze of information for you. Hopefully, what you'll find here is a balanced, practical approach, along with some options to supplement the treatment you may already be receiving. At no point should you ignore conventional treatments such as psychotherapy and antidepressants for severe depression. However, for milder depression, it seems that some viable complementary options are available.

Women Seek Out Integrative Medicine

Alternative medicines may seem new, but they've actually been around for some time. Europeans, for example, have been way ahead of those of us in the United States when it comes to trying the unfamiliar.

Something's happening, though.[1] Women are turning away from traditional doctors and healthcare in large numbers because they feel that they are not getting the effective treatment they need. Instead, they're seeking alternative forms of medicine, especially in areas for which traditional medicine can't always offer a cure. About 65 percent of the market of herbal remedies, vitamins, minerals, and amino acids targets women, and it's working. Women today are more likely than men to take vitamins and minerals, "antiblues" like St. John's wort, SAM-e, resistance-enhancing echinacea and goldenseal, or just go to the spa for a relaxing massage.

This is Dr. Weber here, and I can certainly identify. As I'm writing, I'm sipping Wellness Echinacea tea, and an hour ago I took a capsule of Oscillococcinum to help me fight off a bug that seems to be going around. This morning, while walking with a neighbor, I recommended a tried-and-true remedy of mixing 1/4 teaspoon baking soda with a glass of warm water to fight off the beginnings of a bladder infection. And I'm not alone. Many of the women in my life are looking into or utilizing resources like these, and we share our proven successes with each other. Women also seem to be taking a more active role in partnering with health care providers. They are staying involved in their health care, not just physically, but also mentally and emotionally. Women are also more likely to seek out natural complementary treatment choices for their children and aging parents. They're also increasingly choosing less invasive and more cost-effective approaches, tending to reserve the conventional medical system for emergencies, high-risk pregnancies and illnesses, or for symptoms that are traumatic, persistent, or alarming.

While this clearly is commendable, there is one caution that should be emphasized: When depressed women try to manage their health alone, they may go undiagnosed or untreated by a professional health care provider. As a result, they may suffer needlessly from severe (although treatable) endogenous depressions. It's important to remember that if you choose integrative health care options, it's still vitally important that you have a complete physical exam by your doctor to rule out physiological causes, as well as a complete mental health evaluation if that seems indicated.

Using Complementary Therapies Wisely

When considering a complementary therapy, keep a few things in mind:

1. Complementary Therapies are Not Always Harmless

Complementary medicine and lifestyle therapies such as spirit/mind/body approaches can give you a sense of taking an intentional active role in your own life and health and can minimize difficult side effects caused by conventional medical regimes. Prayer, meditation, relational support, nutritional wellness, exercise, and massage all promote health in general, as well as build resistance and resilience to many illnesses and depression.

On the other hand, some pharmacological, herbal, and even vitamin supplementation can be harmful when overdosed or mixed with other medications. Herbs are God's natural pharmaceuticals, but must be taken wisely. Those who try extreme dietary approaches, for example, are at risk for unhealthy weight loss and nutritional imbalances. Just because a substance or regime seems natural, it doesn't mean that there aren't necessary precautions that need to be observed. For example, you can overdose on St. John's wort, since it has an active ingredient similar to a prescription medication for depression. When taking any remedy, even if it seems harmless, do your homework and be informed. Ask your doctor or another health care professional for information on any complementary medicine and know what the limits and cautions are.

2. It's Important to Research Evidence

Many of the complementary approaches to treatment are still in the process of being researched in the United States. As the evidence for these options is gathered, they will either slowly gain credibility and move into mainstream healthcare (such as mind/body and herbal therapies) or they will be abandoned. Make yourself aware of these studies and controversies surrounding a particular substance and some of the side effects, limitations, and cautions.

Fortunately, new and better research is currently being conducted by the National Institutes of Health (NIH). Some of the controversial substances being researched include Melatonin, St. John's wort, SAM-e, kava, and valerian. In the meantime, it is best to use these cautiously, sticking with the recommended dose and duration.

Where Do I Even Start?

Before utilizing any self-help strategy or complementary therapy, make sure you have a medical checkup. Work in partnership with your health care providers, not against them, and when you explore options for utilizing alternative remedies and a wellness lifestyle, do so with your doctor's approval. If your doctor recommends it, get a complete mental health evaluation, and from there, cooperate with the recommended treatment plan. Discuss these complementary and alternative options with the professional help you are getting, but do not try to treat depression on your own.

In addition, do your homework. When looking at research, look for that which has been done on humans, not just animals. In addition to talking to your doctor, go to a bookstore or look for information on the Internet. Make sure the resources you're relying on are valid and backed up by solid organizations, health care professionals, and research that is referenced. Remember: When you do research on the web, you may come across unreliable information. In general, medically oriented and university-based sites will provide the most trustworthy information. For further resource ideas, see the resource section in the back of this book.

There Are Alternatives

In a moment, we'll look at a few natural remedies for depression and related disorders in detail. But there's something else we should cover first. Although antidepressant medications are often necessary for the treatment of depression, natural supplements can be helpful, as well—as long as they're taken with the approval of your doctor. In some cases, alternative treatments could be the best prescription of all. Consider, for example, someone whose liver doesn't function correctly. Since the liver helps dispose of antidepressant medications once they've done their work, a healthy liver is essential. Alternative natural remedies may be an option—though it's still important to check with your doctor first. That "natural" substance may need to be disposed of through the liver, as well.

There may be other reasons why you can't take antidepressants or tolerate the side effects, and in those cases, a natural remedy may be worth considering, too. For those women who experience chronic mild depression or PMS mood swings, natural remedies—along with a healthy lifestyle—may be just what the doctor ordered.

Herbal Antidepressants and Complementary Medicines

"Their fruit will be for food, and their leaves for medicine" (Ezek. 47:12, NASB).

". . . and the leaves of the tree were for the healing of the nations" (Rev. 22:2, NASB).

St. John's Wort (Hypericum Perforatum)

St. John's wort has been used in traditional herbal medicine for centuries, primarily for wound healing. As the tale goes, "wort" is Old English for "plant." St. John's wort was named for John the Baptist, whose birthday, June 24, supposedly falls around the time this plant, growing in the wild, produces its yellow flowers.

For the many millions of women who experience mild to moderate depression, who feel stress associated with depression, who are concerned about the side effects of antidepressants, or who suffer from seasonal affective disorder or chronic, low-grade unhappiness (dysthymia), St. John's wort has become a readily available, natural antidepressant option that can relieve these depressions. In some primary care settings, leading physicians like Dr. Isadore Rosenfeld begin treatment by prescribing St. John's wort for mild depression. In other conventional settings, there is still caution about its use, as many await the outcome of further research.

The National Institute of Mental Health, in collaboration with the NIH Office of Alternative Medicine (OAM) and the NIH Office of Dietary Supplements (ODS), recently launched a three-year, $4.3 million study that included 336 people with major depression, conducted at thirteen clinical sites across the U.S. This was the first large-scale, controlled clinical trial in the United States to assess whether St. John's wort has significant therapeutic effectiveness in treating clinical depression.[2]

Also, recently after reviewing over 30 clinical trials on St. John's wort, the Council for Responsible Nutrition declared that it is safe and beneficial for mild to moderate depression, stress, and anxiety.

How St. John's Wort Works

Experts still don't exactly know how St. John's wort works, so it's considered an "atypical" antidepressant. While it is still being researched, new explanations are continually being advanced.

Basically, experts believe St. John's wort may affect many neurotransmitters and chemicals. It seems that many ingredients work together for a broader benefit, unlike that found in synthetic antidepressants.[3]

In summary, St. John's wort has complex effects and works within the central nervous system to correct chemical imbalances that may lead to depression.

Possible Side Effects

About 2.5 percent of people taking St. John's wort may experience mild side effects including: gastrointestinal irritation, nausea, indigestion, abdominal pains, dry mouth, dizziness, fatigue, and increased sensitivity to light. St. John's wort has also been recently linked to formation of cataracts with long-term use. This means that a natural substance like St. John's wort is not immune from side-effects, and should be used with full awareness of its risks.

Cautions When Taking St. John's Wort

St. John's wort can have the same side effects as many medications that are prescribed for depression, and should not be taken together with any of the conventional medications as it could increase serotonin levels to a toxic level. That's known as a serotonin crisis, and requires emergency room help. While taking St. John's wort, avoid prolonged exposure to sunlight, especially if you have fair skin. In addition, avoid foods containing tyramine (such as cheese and red wine), alcohol, narcotics, amphetamines, cold remedies, and antidepressant drugs. Have your blood pressure checked every week or two, as it could be elevated. St. John's wort can also prolong the sedating effects of anesthetics and can reduce the concentration of anticoagulants (blood thinners like aspirin) and oral contraceptives.

Kava Root (Piper Methysticum)

Some researchers consider the kava root as a treatment alternative to tranquilizers and synthetic antidepressants for anxiety disorders. And since many depressions are accompanied by anxiety, it only makes sense to mention it here. Kava reduces anxiety without causing lethargy or the "fuzzy brain" often associated with synthetic tranquilizers such as Xanax. This herb, from the black pepper family, is also thought to help alleviate migraine headaches and menstrual cramps.

Researchers are not completely clear on how kava works. Some theorize that it has a direct soothing action on an overactive amygdala, which is the brain's alarm center, thus relieving anxiety and elevating mood. Many studies have been done with patients suffering from anxiety, agoraphobia, specific phobias, and social phobias, and showed that they were helped in the areas of anxiety, fear, tension, and insomnia. They also steadily improved with treatment.

The recommended dosage is 45 to 100 mg kavalactones three times a day. For insomnia, take 200 to 300 mg before bed. Kava can be taken with St. John's wort.

Cautions When Taking Kava

Consuming kava on a daily basis is not recommended for longer than twenty-five weeks, or four to six months. When taken in small amounts on an occasional basis, it can be used longer, if necessary. If 85 mg three times a day is not reducing your anxiety, then see a doctor for another evaluation and consider a stronger prescription drug.

Kava should not be taken at all if

- you're already taking a benzodiazepine tranquilizer such as Xanax, as it could cause disorientation and lethargy;
- you're suffering from Parkinson's disease, as it could worsen muscular twitching;
- you've been drinking alcohol;
- you're taking pharmaceutical antidepressants, benzodiazepine tranquilizers, sleeping pills, or any other

prescription medication and haven't checked with your doctor;

- you're driving or operating heavy machinery;
- you're pregnant or breastfeeding; or
- it's the only remedy you're using for a severe anxiety disorder or severe depression. See a doctor.

Ginkgo Biloba

Ginkgo improves blood supply to the brain and improves mental functioning. It has been used as an aid in stroke recovery, mental acuity, and Alzheimer's disease in elderly people. It also appears to normalize neurotransmitter levels, and is considered to be an antidepressant due to its apparent serotonin-enhancing effect.

The recommended dosage of ginkgo biloba is 40 to 80 mg two or three times a day. Ginkgo can also be taken with St. John's wort.

Cautions When Taking Ginkgo

Don't use more than 240 mg a day, or you may develop diarrhea, restlessness, and irritability. Those taking aspirin or other blood thinners should also avoid ginkgo.

Valerian Root

Valerian root *(Valeriana officinalis)* is a popular herbal medicine that has been called the Valium and mood stabilizer alternative. Despite its awful smell, (like dirty socks or something rotten), valerian is becoming the most widely used sleeping sedative. Throughout the world, it has gained popularity for its ability to calm anxiety, nervousness, high-anxiety depression, and relieve insomnia. In many clinical studies, valerian has repeatedly been shown to reduce the amount of time it takes to fall asleep and to increase the quality of sleep among poor sleepers, smokers, and heavy coffee drinkers. During World War I, it was used to calm the shell-shocked soldiers and continues to be used to calm people under stress and for those with generalized anxiety, depression, and insomnia. The recommended dosage is 300 to 900 mg (0.8 percent valeric acid) before bedtime. To reduce performance anxiety or stress, take 50 to 100 mg two or three times a day.

Cautions When Taking Valerian

Valerian has a long history of safety, but as it is somewhat of a sedative, it is advisable to avoid drinking and operating heavy machinery after taking it and to be careful when driving. It is not addicting. There are generally no side effects, but in rare cases headaches and paradoxical stimulant-type effects such as nervousness, restlessness, agitation, and palpitations have been reported. Valerian should not be taken nightly for longer than six months at a time, as it may become toxic or a depressant.

Uplifting Amino Acids

SAM-e (S-Adenosyl-Methionine)

SAM-e, pronounced "sammy," is expected to revolutionize the treatment of depression in the United States as it has for two decades in Europe, according to the authors of *Stop Depression Now*.[4] This acclaimed team from Columbia University and Baylor University have been studying SAM-e for fifteen years. SAM-e appears comparable to state-of-the-art treatments for depression and arthritis. Unlike the leading drug therapies, however, it doesn't have significant side effects. According to Dr. Richard Brown, SAM-e is the best anti-depressant he's ever prescribed, and is cheaper than many prescription remedies. Since SAM-e was introduced into the United States in March 1999, it has become a safe, over-the-counter, natural supplement that promises to help you beat depression quickly, easily, and safely. Many psychiatrists are endorsing the use of Sam-e in cases of mild to moderate depression.

Besides St. John's wort, SAM-e is perhaps the next most studied and utilized nonpharmaceutical depression remedy, and many predict it will eventually outsell St. John's wort. It is most effective in treating retarded depressions, such as those marked by lethargy, apathy, guilt, and suicidal impulses, as well as for seasonal affective disorder, postpartum depression, menopausal mood swings, PMS, sleep disturbances, and subsyndromal depressions known as "the blues."[5]

How SAM-e Works

SAM-e is not an herb, drug, or vitamin. It is a substance that is already in your body. Normally the brain manufactures all the SAM-e it needs from the amino acid methionine and adenosine triphosphate, a molecular energy source. However, SAM-e synthesis gets impaired and shows lower levels in those who are depressed.[6]

Supplementing the diet with SAM-e results in increased levels of serotonin and dopamine and improved binding of neurotransmitters to receptor sites. This causes increased serotonin and dopamine activity and improved brain cell membrane fluidity, resulting in significant improvement in your mood.

Side Effects

Some users have experienced mild mania effects such as with other antidepressants. A few have also reported hot, itchy ears as a side effect.[7]

A dosage of 200 mg twice a day to start is recommended, as higher doses may cause nausea and vomiting. After a few days, dosage can increase to 400 mg twice a day. A few days later, increase again to three times a day.

Cautions When Taking SAM-e

Those experiencing bipolar (manic) depression should not take SAM-e, due to its susceptibility to provoking hypomania or mania. This effect is already experienced by some with bipolar depression.

Serotonin Boosters: Tryptophan and 5-HTP

L-tryptophan is the metabolic precursor of serotonin and melatonin, neurotransmitters with sedative qualities that are useful in the treatment of depression symptoms. However, L-tryptophan has been banned in the United States due to an incidence of contamination. A newly available supplement, 5-hydroxytryptamine (5-HTP) is now available. Studies show that 5-HTP is biochemically closer to serotonin, chemically known as 5-hydroxytryptamine, and elevates beta-endorphins, the "feel good" hormones. 5-HTP is the intermediate between tryptophan and serotonin.

5-HTP can work for all varieties and severities of depression. It is particularly well-suited for melancholic and treatment-resistant major depressions, since these typically are associated with high levels of the stress hormone cortisol, which lowers blood levels of tryptophan.

The recommended dosage is 200 mg a day.

Omega-3 Fatty Acids

In some women suffering from depression, there is a clear association between depression and a diet lacking in sufficient omega-3 fatty acids. American diets seem to be deficient in omega-3 fatty polyunsaturated fatty acids, which are necessary for proper nerve functioning, and that has a direct impact on mental functioning. Low-fat diets have especially caused this damage, depriving the body of necessary "good" fats. Omega-3 fatty acids are integral components of the brain's cellular membranes, including the crucial synapses where neurons exchange chemical signals. Nerve cell membranes in the brain are protected by DHA, a long chain of omega-3 fatty acids. Adequate amounts of DHA ensure optimal composition of nerve cell membranes in the brain.

Low levels of omega-3 also influence the action of monomine oxidase, the enzyme responsible for breaking down serotonin, epinephrine, and dopamine.

The best sources of omega-3 fatty acids are cold water fish like salmon and halibut, eaten one or two times a week. You can also take it in supplement form as fish oil or flaxseed oil. A great source is Spectrum Essentials' Organic Flax Oil, available in health food stores either cold pressed or in capsules. You can also sprinkle flax seeds on your cereal, or buy flax seed frozen waffles.

Nutritional Supplements

Certain vitamin deficiencies have also been linked to depression. This could be due to factors like food fads that lead to medical conditions, alcoholism, poor absorption of nutrients in the intestine, nerve cell deficiencies due to medication, or the fact that the body simply can't absorb nutrients correctly. Nutritional deficiencies of things like vitamin B or folic acid can cause feelings of apathy, depression, insomnia, irritability, nervousness, personality changes, lowered mental function, or confusion, as well as reduce your response to medicinal therapies. Antidepressant medication is also less effective if there are low levels of B vitamins and folic acid. Raising them to standard measures can not only help relieve depression, but can also make antidepressants work better. Several studies have shown that as many as 80 percent of depressed people have low levels of vitamin B6 and serotonin.[8] Deficiencies of vitamin B6 can cause your nerve cells to reduce the amount of serotonin availability, an important brain neurotransmitter involved in depression. Another common deficiency in the United States that has been linked to depression is vitamin B12. It is easily destroyed in cooking and is an underconsumed food group found in leafy green vegetables.

Eat a Well-Balanced Diet and Take Supplements

Focus on eating a well-balanced diet, including plenty of leafy greens such as spinach, brewer's yeast, avocados, and orange juice for folic acid. For vitamin B6, eat bananas, avocados, dark leafy greens, chicken, greens, legumes, fish, and whole grains. Foods rich in vitamin B12, on the other hand, include high protein choices like oysters, tuna, yogurt, milk, and chicken. These will not only make you less depressed, but will also have a moderate and lasting effect on brain chemistry, mood, and energy level. They will also keep you from craving too much of the refined foods you shouldn't eat.

A number of minerals play a role in contributing to or preventing depression, irritability, and mood swings, and they include calcium, iron, magnesium, selenium, and zinc. Low levels of magnesium can result in personality changes, weakness, and poor concentration. Stress also stimulates hormones, which, in turn, increases magnesium loss from the cells. To boost levels of magnesium in your body, consider eating a banana at breakfast and a dark-green salad with almonds at lunch. Take a magnesium supplement of 400 mg a day to ensure depression symptom relief. To get adequate vitamins and minerals in your diet, a high-potency supplement formula is suggested. In addition, consider the following supplements:

Vitamin B complex with:
    Vitamin B6 100 mg
    Vitamin B12 800 mcg per day
    Folic acid 800 mcg per day
Vitamin C 500 to 1,000 mg three times a day
Vitamin E 200 to 400 IU per day
Omega-3 fatty acids—Flaxseed oil 1 tablespoon per day
Calcium 250 mg three times a day
Magnesium 250 mg three times a day or 400 mg per day

Also, as needed:

5-HTP 100 mg three times per day or
SAM-e 400 mg twice a day[9]

Light Therapy

Those who live in dark climates without enough sunlight often suffer from a form of depression called seasonal affective disorder, or SAD. For some, this disorder doesn't need a very dark winter, just a very cloudy one. The reason for such depression is fairly well understood, and it all revolves around a brain hormone called melatonin, which plays a major role in controlling a daily or circadian rhythm. For both animals and humans, melatonin is released in the brain with the onset of darkness. In animals it controls hibernation and activity levels.

Since the problem in this type of depression is an insufficiency of light, it only makes sense that the remedy would be light therapy.

With this type of therapy, depressed people sit under artificial light approximating sunlight for extended periods, usually several hours a day, and the depression is relieved.

Many SAD sufferers can benefit from taking morning walks outside. Others vacation in sunny places to break the persistent subdued exposure to darkness. Some spend a week or two in a sunny place just before the onset of winter and "step up" their exposure to sunlight. And others have installed light rooms in their homes.

Perhaps all depression sufferers should consider increasing their outdoor activities. Not only will it ensure that your melatonin system is properly reset on a daily basis, but exercise and other healthy habits and interventions have proven to be good for relieving depression as well.

Music Therapy

This is Dr. Webber here, and as I write this, I am listening to music that has been designed to relax the body while keeping the mind alert. For years, experts in audiology, psychology, medicine, education, human development, psychoacoustics, and music have researched the powerful effect music can have on mood and emotions. The healing power of using "music as medicine" has been utilized for centuries.[10] Music has been designed for thinking, learning, improving concentration, and increasing productivity, for relaxing and for destressing. Think, for example, of wonderful orchestral arrangements mixed with nature sounds.

God created music for us to enjoy, to soothe and "massage" our nervous systems, and to uplift our spirits. In the

Bible, Saul's distress could only be soothed and refreshed by David's worship on the lyre. Today, hospitals, institutions, and even jails use music to lift people's moods, ease pain, and break through the walls of isolation. Music can even lessen the level of stress hormones, blood pressure, respiratory rate, and stomach and intestinal contractions.

Daily listening to music ought to be an important part of your wellness healing plan. When feeling down and depressed, you can choose music that is uplifting, nurturing, and inspiring to you, especially praise and worship. For some, happy, loud music can be annoying. Instead, you may identify with music written by others who have suffered, or old hymns. If you feel stressed, choose music that will soothe, relax, or inspire you. In the evening when getting ready for bed, listen to music that will calm you and prepare you for a good night's sleep.

Stress Reduction Relaxation Techniques

Stress can be reduced in a variety of ways. Here's a start.

Deep Breathing

Have you heard the saying, "Stop, take a deep breath, and count to ten?" This is actually a very useful and effective way of managing stressful situations. When stressed, one of the negative physiological responses is that breathing becomes shallow and rapid. Deep breathing can reduce your body's stress response and help calm your mind. When feeling stressed during the day, take a few minutes to sit or stand comfortably and do some deep breathing. Starting and ending your day this way is also a good idea.

Inhale slowly and deeply through the nose and count to ten. Expand your diaphragm and fill your lungs completely. Exhale through the nose slowly and completely, also counting to ten. Concentrate on the breathing and counting through each cycle. You'll notice that your body will relax, and your mind will become more focused and quiet. Repeat this deep breathing cycle at least five times, and as needed when you feel stressed.

Progressive Muscle Relaxation

Muscle relaxation techniques, along with deep breathing, are quite effective when it comes to relaxing and falling asleep. When done once or twice a day, for at least ten minutes, stress and anxiety can be greatly reduced. This method has been widely researched and proven effective. In this technique, you contract a set of major muscles to experience tension, then gradually relax them until they're completely loose. When in this intentional relaxed state, the physical system cannot be stressed or anxious.

To practice progressive muscle relaxation, find a quiet, comfortable place. Lie on your back with your arms along the sides of your body and your eyes closed. You will progressively move throughout the body, tightening a group of muscles and feeling the tightness, then letting go and feeling the relaxation. Begin with your arms. First clench the left fist, feel the tightness, and then let go. Feel the relaxation in the muscles of the left hand. Now go to the right fist and do the same. Move to the left arm, then the right arm, and then both arms, each time tightening the muscles and letting go. Then proceed to the left foot, the right foot, and then the lower legs and upper legs, one at a time, doing the progressive muscle relaxation for each muscle group. Move to the face. Wrinkle the forehead by lifting the eyebrows. Feel the tightness, then let go and relax. Progressively do each part of the face this way, first by dropping the eyebrows and frowning, then closing the eyes tightly shut, clenching the jaw, and finally, tightening the lips then relaxing. Next, bend the neck forward, tighten and relax, and then do the exercise rotating the neck to the right, then to the left. Move to the shoulders, the trunk of the body, and the stomach. Again, for each muscle group, tighten and relax. Stay with the relaxed feeling for a few minutes before completing the exercise. Try doing this progressive muscle relaxation technique for twenty to thirty minutes a day as a great way to reduce the accumulative damaging effects of stress in your life.

Meditation

By meditation, we are referring to a Christian approach to meditation, not to Eastern religious forms of meditation. David meditated day and night on God's Word, and we are encouraged to "meditate" or focus our mind on things that will result in right living and God's peace (Phil. 4:8). As Christians, we can also learn how to effectively meditate through what science and research has discovered about the physiological and mental values of meditation.

God's design for meditation is to quiet and relax the mind, focus thoughts on things that are positive, beautiful, hopeful, and not stress-provoking. Meditation blocks thoughts that produce stress and anxiety, thereby calming the mind and body. Successful meditation, which results in deep relaxation, can be very energizing. This is complementary to deep breathing and progressive relaxation, which relax the body. Done regularly, you can also reduce the physiological effects of stress and anxiety and attain more peace by experiencing a reduction in heart rate, blood pressure, and adrenaline levels. Meditation alone has been found to be more effective in reducing blood pressure and anxiety than muscle relaxation, since it calms both the body and the mind.

Begin your day with a twenty-minute "quiet" meditation time. This can be done in a variety of ways, but the main idea is to focus, concentrating your thoughts and attention on a particular theme from God's Word, God, or Jesus himself, and away from your own wandering thoughts, stresses, worries, or anxieties. When your mind wanders, bring it back to the central point you were focusing on. If distracting thoughts persist, write them down so you can refer to them at a later time.

Throughout the day, you can continue the benefits of this kind of focus through techniques such as mini-meditations, or practicing the presence of God. Focus on the here and now. Through the use of your senses, heighten your awareness of God's presence with you and your immediate surrounding environment. For example, stop and smell the roses. Breathe in the smell deeply and focus on the beauty God has created. Thank him for all he has created and all his goodness to you. Even in the mundane, while washing the dishes, you can concentrate on the feel of the water on your hands, being aware of all your immediate sensory experiences in the kitchen: touch, smell, color. If your mind wanders, redirect your brain from your stressful thoughts and worries to pleasant senses, and that will disrupt the stress adaptation response and evoke relaxation.

A caution regarding relaxation and meditation to those women who are depressed. If you are severely depressed, and not agitated, it is not recommended that you try these techniques; your automatic nervous system may not need to be lowered any further, and your depression may actually be aggravated.

PART 4

Strategies for Overcoming Depression

10

Strategies
for Recovery

> My inner self waits earnestly for you, Lord; you are my
> help and shield, for in you my heart rejoices, because I
> have trusted and been confident in your holy name.
> Let your mercy and loving kindness, O Lord, be upon me
> in proportion to my waiting and hoping for you.
>
> Prayer inspired by Psalm 33:16, 18–22

Any journey is easier with a road map, and the trek from depression to recovery is no different. Without a plan, you can easily find yourself lost—and in this case, missing some effective strategies for reaching the "ultimate destination" of total healing.

Before beginning your journey, however, a "briefing" is in order to give you some inside tips and insight into what lies ahead. Remember: Many have gone before you on the journey to recovery, and you can learn from their experience. If certain strategies have worked for others as they've struggled to get out of their depression quagmire, it's likely that these strategies will work for you, too. You might even be able to avoid their mistakes.

In previous chapters, we outlined a number of strategies for treating and dealing with depression. Next, we'll talk about what you can do for yourself. It's truly a more comprehensive approach, and both must go together.

Consider this, then, your briefing, a chance for us to encourage you and lay a foundation upon which all the other strategies on your journey toward overcoming depression depend. You can take all the medication in the world or do a lifetime's worth of therapy, but unless you pay attention to the strategies we outline here, you may still fall right back into depression. We will also provide some basic guidelines for developing a practical set of lifestyle strategies.

Basic Strategies for Overcoming Depression

1. Admit You Are Struggling with Depression

Perhaps the greatest obstacle to recovery, as in all of life's struggles, is the refusal to own up to the struggle. We call this denial. It's always an obstacle to healing.

Some of you may struggle with depression symptoms that you have not yet recognized and admitted, and the people around you don't know, either. You might think you're "coping" or getting through it all right. But the more you deny your depression, the more it will progress, until you become withdrawn and isolated.

Admittedly, it is difficult to know when to heed the warning signs of depression, especially in the early stages. Our tendency, especially if we are busy, is to just ignore them and hope they will go away. Also, because women experience many ups and downs, far more than men, they can't always tell when their depression is normal and when it requires professional help. They may feel many aches and pains, not sleep well, feel "off" and tired, stressed, frustrated in relationships, and "stuck," but not realize that these could all be symptoms of depression. Unfortunately, as time goes on and the signs of depression become more debilitating, it gets more difficult to tell the difference between what is "you," what is "your fault" or "weakness," and what the best plan of action is for getting better.

So, if you recognize any of the symptoms of depression in your life, it is important to admit to yourself that you are depressed and do something about it.

2. Be Honest and Open with God in Prayer

It is vitally important that you build in time to talk with and listen to God and to openly and honestly express your thoughts and feelings with him. Tell God about your spiritual confusion, disappointments, even anger at him if you feel it. He can handle it; he already knows that you feel this way. Let God be with you in your feelings, thoughts, and experience.

What God is longing for, and what you need on an ongoing basis, is a deeper relationship with him. Ask him to show you the underlying causes of your depression and to direct you to the right people to support you and where you should go for professional help. Ask him to search your heart and heal you. Ask for strength and courage to make the healthy choices that will continue to give you healing.

When you call on God for help with your longings and desires, admitting your deep needs and where you've fallen short, he hears you. He has promised that as you call out to him, he will lighten your load and give his Holy Spirit to heal, comfort, and strengthen you. Meet with other believers in prayer, Bible study, encouraging teaching, and uplifting worship.

3. Share Your Struggles with Someone Who Is Going to Be Supportive and Empathic

Once you have acknowledged your depression to yourself and God, tell one or more trusted people in your life about it, as well. It can be your husband, but tell a few women in your life, as well, such as your mother, sister, or close friends. Tell them that you are struggling and that you are depressed. Ask them if they will be with you, allow you to talk when you need to, help you think through what you should do, and help you figure out who to see for professional guidance.

Women who have overcome difficult times say that the connections they have with women relatives and friends in their lives were crucial in getting them through the journey of overcoming depression, as well as other life struggles. I have often heard women say, "I couldn't have made it without my women friends (or my mother, or sisters). They prayed with me and for me, and their just 'being there' for me was a life saver." Women regularly need other women who they can be brutally honest with about their feelings and problems, including how lousy they feel.

For some of you, depression may be linked to struggles in your marriage. The marriage may be okay overall, but maybe you go up and down emotionally, depending on how the little things aggravate your relationship. Without violating or betraying confidence with your husband, you have to be able to debrief with other women and "tell it like it is" in your life and marriage. This is especially important for those of you who are Christian leaders, therapists, and other caregivers. It is difficult to share with others that you're miserable or fighting with your husband. But choose one or more trusted women to share your heart with, and you will experience the benefits, as many other women do, of the "lightening of your load," by externalizing and verbalizing your feelings and receiving empathy and encouragement.

4. Create Meaningful Connections

Build healthy connections. We have emphasized this several times, and we want to reiterate it here. You need one or more significant relationships where you can meet regularly and talk, but not necessarily about your depression. You need a broad range of friends. Many women say that this is what gets them through the hard times. These friends, like the people in an adult Sunday school group or a woman's group, will help you to maintain perspective and give you the encouragement you need to keep going. These are women friends with whom you can be genuine, but not necessarily intimate, and who will be empathic with you.

One of the symptoms of depression is a tendency to withdraw and isolate from others. So, getting together with other women may take some effort and some commitment on your part, but by doing it, you help to relieve this symptom. Get regularly scheduled times set in place that don't require frequent phone calls to arrange. Many such groups are available to you if you are connected to a church, such as prayer groups, small groups, walking or jogging partners, or prayer partners. If you are not connected to a church, then become connected right away.

We all need meaningful connections with one another, including friends, family, neighbors, community, and church. We also need to connect and reconnect with God and ourselves about our past, our traditions, and our hopes and visions for the future. These connections are what give us meaning in life, as well as physical health and even longevity.

5. Learn to Feel and Express Your Emotions

Our emotions have been called the "eyes and ears" of our hearts, and they can help us find our bearings and give us a sense of who we are. God created it that way. So becoming aware of your feelings and expressing them in healthy ways is a key strategy in overcoming depression emotionally.

It's very common for women who are depressed to fear feelings. You fear falling apart, being consumed by your emotions, and are afraid that if you start crying, you'll never stop. However, there is nothing to fear about emotions, except the fear itself. While depressed, the chemicals released in your brain influence thought, which impacts your emotions, which influences your interaction with others.

Some positive emotions like love, hope, and joy will be dampened. This is called anhedonia, meaning that you have lost your ability to experience any form of pleasure. On the other hand, the negative emotions, guilt, anger, diminished self-esteem, etc., will be increased. This is an interesting effect of depression.

Choosing a safe place to express your feelings can actually help lift a depressed mood, at least temporarily. So, tell God how you feel, have a good cry, call a friend, journal your feelings, talk to a therapist, or feel your feelings through listening to music, playing an instrument, or engaging some other creative art expression. It all helps.

If you struggle with unresolved emotional challenges from early trauma, anger, hurt, loss, unforgiveness, or bitterness, or if you're not able to get in touch with your primary emotions, consider professional counseling. A counselor can help you feel your emotions in a healthy way and constructively walk you through the healing process.

6. Allow Yourself Some "Down" Times

Be patient and kind to yourself. There will be days you will need to take time to allow yourself to cry, grieve, and process the depression. Don't feel like this is wasted time. Let yourself go with the flow of your feelings.

In addition, structure balance in your life so that you are with people and able to get things done, so you don't get stuck being isolated and overwhelmed with the low feelings.

7. Commit to Going All the Way through the Valley of Depression

You can't fight against depression; you have to learn to cooperate with it. It is important to keep the balance of being intentional and responsibly allowing for some down time, as well as time when you override your depression and do what must be done. Depression is a powerful force that interferes with everyday functioning and enjoyment. It can trigger physical illness and leave you feeling negative, helpless, and hopeless. As we mentioned earlier, it is important to allow yourself time out to cry, grieve, process your feelings, read, or just watch movies. However, don't stay in this place of withdrawal, or, as men like to call it, "the cave." You can stay in such a place too long, suffering and brewing on negative thoughts. Set a time limit. Use a kitchen timer if you like. Allow yourself ten or twenty minutes, and when the time is up, return to action and take an active role in nurturing, caring for, changing, and renewing yourself. Get all the help you need through counseling, social support, and medication when necessary.

Ultimately it will require courage to persevere and to allow God to mature you through this season. We want to encourage you to keep going. Every day is a new day, and a new opportunity to get closer to your recovery. Don't give up!

8. Set Small Goals and Take Small Steps

Set goals and priorities for yourself, but don't be unrealistic. Don't try to do it all, only to add defeat and discouragement. Do what you can. Start with a small, manageable goal or task for the day or the week, one that you can accomplish. Break down tasks into smaller, doable parts. You have control over the here and now. Don't expect too much of yourself too soon, as you will set yourself up for defeat. Don't be afraid to try something different; learning new skills, implementing healthy lifestyle choices, can help bring recovery. But take one step at a time.

9. Remember, Growing and Changing Happens One Day at a Time

It was Charlie Brown who said, "I've developed a new philosophy . . . I only dread one day at a time."

Knowing all the facts and theories about depression will not be enough to heal you; there are also daily steps that must be taken toward growth and wellness. Recovery from depression takes time. It may be weeks before you see improvement, so don't get discouraged. Also, try not to be overwhelmed by all that is expected of you. No doubt many of our depressed readers are feeling overwhelmed right now with all of this information. All you have to remember is to start with one area of your life today and then take it a day at a time. Don't try to remember every bit of advice we or anyone else may be giving you. Grasp on to one idea that is helpful and go with that. You can always go back and reread what we have written. That's the beauty of a book, after all; it's always there for you!

If the idea of self-nurture, care, growth, and a wellness lifestyle are new to you, just focus on one small part of change. You may need to experiment and find what works for you. And you only have to do it one day at a time.

10. Make Good Use of Your "Up" Times

As your treatment starts to take effect, you will experience brief periods when you feel good again. Unfortunately, in the early stages, those times may not last. Eventually, though, these good periods will get longer and longer until they stay permanently.

In the meantime, make good use of the times you feel better, no matter how short-lived. When you do have a good day, a reprieve from your symptoms, use the restored energy to do something to nurture yourself or to catch up on the chores that have been neglected. It will help you feel better and raise your hope. You might even notice there are certain times of the day that you feel better, so use these to your advantage. Do some menu planning; look through magazines for recipes or ideas; take time to exercise; meet with a friend and do something fun that you enjoy. Be sure to journal these good times, as your doctor will want to know about them. Write down the new discoveries you are making, the changes in your feelings and thinking, what's helping, and what strategies are worth repeating. Write an encouraging note to yourself to read when you might feel down again.

11. Avoid Making Major Life Decisions until the Depression Lifts

It is a big mistake to trust your judgment while you are in depression. In other words, don't make any life decisions about yourself, your children, or your family until you are stable mentally, emotionally, spiritually, and physically. Remember, depression distorts emotions and thinking which pass once the depression lifts.

12. Get the Help You Need

As we have covered in the previous chapters, it is vitally important that you get a physical examination to rule out medical causes for your depression. Also be open to considering professional counseling and taking an antidepressant if recommended. Remember: Get help as soon as you can. The longer you wait, the harder it gets, and the longer it will take for your recovery.

13. Learn All You Can about Depression

Educate yourself about depression by learning and reading on the topic. By reading this book, you are already enriching your healing process. Keep up on the latest developments in treatment and be encouraged by other women's stories of recovery. The more you know about depression, the less helpless you will feel about not being able to control it. You will become more empowered and hopeful, as well as gain direction to develop a strategy for your recovery.

Strategies for Wellness Living

One of the most difficult things to do when you're depressed is to take good care of yourself. You don't feel like doing your favorite things, or much of anything. You could land up isolating yourself, being drawn to foods that are bad for you, not sleep well, not exercise, get caught in the downward spiral of negative thinking, and feel spiritually dry and dejected by God. There usually isn't much energy left to care for yourself, and so the necessary self-care for your healing must be intentional. Depression impacts those around you, at work and at home. Investing in your own health and healing is the very key to your healing and the heart of your home. So, don't feel guilty for taking time for yourself. Our doctors' orders are for you to give yourself permission to be aware of your symptoms of depression, get the help you need, start developing a strategy for your healing, and take good care of yourself. In addition to getting the support and professional help you need that we've covered so far, we would also like to remind you of some practical basics for a healthy lifestyle that are essential to your recovery as a whole person. Although these might sound very simple, don't underestimate how crucial daily choices and habits are to a more effective and lasting recovery. And please don't be overwhelmed. Start with the area that you are having the most difficulty with, and then slowly address the others.

1. Your Food Does Affect Your Mood

There is a connection between your depression, your brain, and the food you put into your mouth. Eat well-balanced, nutritious mini-meals. It's important to keep your blood levels steady and to supply your body with the necessary nutrients. We went into this in more detail in the chapter on natural complementary therapy. Remember, certain vitamin deficiencies have been linked to depression. When your appetite is down and you don't eat regularly, and you reach for refined sweets, junk food, and caffeine, these all play a part in the onset, severity, and duration of depression. So be sure to help lift those depleted serotonin levels by eating frequent small meals (at least three, and up to five, mini-meals), drinking plenty of water (at least eight glasses), and eating a balanced diet with plenty of fresh fruits and vegetables. In addition, include whole grains, as well as lean proteins rich in tryptophan, such as turkey, chicken, fish, milk, bananas, peanuts, and lentils.

2. Get Adequate Sleep

Another symptom associated with depression, stress, and anxiety is sleep disturbances. Being exhausted can also lead to depression. So, getting enough sleep is key to your recovery. It's hard to battle the negative effects of stress and debilitating symptoms of depression—not to mention "being like Jesus"—when you're tired and exhausted. Sleep refreshes and restores the body, mind, and emotions, as well as uplifts the spirit. Get at least eight hours of sleep a night. Take naps during the day if needed.

3. Physical Activity Is "Mood-Boosting"

A growing number of studies shows that exercise has been found to be an effective, mood-boosting natural antidepressant treatment for depression. Brisk walking or jogging for thirty minutes a day, at least three to four times a week, can actually treat depression as well as medication. Basically, aerobic exercise releases a variety of cortisone-type hormones that can lighten the symptoms of depression. Exercise increases levels of endorphins, the body's own mood-elevating natural antidepressants, as well as boosts levels of serotonin, which alleviates depression. Physical activity also helps you sleep better, improves your appetite, and raises your sexual desire. Choose a physical activity you enjoy, be patient, and stick with it. You will eventually notice results and will not want to miss a day.

4. Reduce Stress

As we discussed at length in the earlier chapter on stress, anxiety, and depression, be mindful of the chronic strain in your life, what is stressful to you, and what could be contributing to your depression or hindering your recovery. Explore the most effective techniques for you for passive and active stress reduction. To those of you who thrive on adrenaline and stress, it's time to learn the importance of lowering your stress response, before the damage is not reversible. Refer to the stress chapter for more guidelines.

5. Journal

Personal, reflective journaling, which involves putting your deepest feelings and thoughts down on paper, has tremendous healing value, emotionally, physically, and spiritually. Studies have shown that those who regularly write in a journal have 30 percent fewer visits to the doctor. When you write, you help relieve yourself of physical and emotional pain, reducing the stress that causes headaches, high blood pressure, and depression. Journal writing can also give you a sense of control and understanding to the situation. When you journal, be honest about your feelings, frustrations, fears, and thoughts. Remember, the journal is only for you. Write whatever comes to your mind, also putting images into words. Balance out expressing your feelings with God's truth and promises to you, what you sense he is saying to you, along with what you are learning. After journaling for a while, you will discover new insights, which contribute to your healing. As you reflect back and read over these, you will see how you have grown and how God has brought you through.

6. Surround Yourself with Positives

One of the causes and symptoms of depression is pessimistic, distorted thinking and ruminating. So, many of you are probably facing a battle of the mind. Thankfully, this way of thinking can be combated and changed. It happens when you learn to dispute the distorted, pessimistic, habitual beliefs and replace them with Biblical, reality-based, optimistic alternatives. If this is a challenge for you, counseling could be helpful in walking you through the process. Practically, on a daily basis, start being aware of surrounding yourself with positives that will counteract your negative thinking and feelings. Choose to be around positive people, events, media, music, and literature.

Seriously, laughter also helps with healing. Laughter is medicine for the soul. Laughter is like internal jogging, allowing the body to release endorphins (that feel good and are calming) to compensate for the stress and strain in your life. So find what tickles your funny bone, like renting a funny movie or reading the humorous cards at the drug store and have a good belly-aching laugh!

Here are some other suggestions of practical ways to positively stimulate your senses that have been meaningful to other women. Try some and, of course, add your own.

- Enjoy the smell of fresh-baked bread and coffee first thing in the morning.
- Burn fragrant candles while working around the house.
- Play uplifting music—Christmas, Celtic, praise and worship.
- Drink flavored teas (like Mango-Passion).
- Bake cookies or a cake and eat some while they are fresh. Share with someone who would also enjoy them.

- Enjoy a "spa" night at home. Take a hot bath by candlelight using fragrant body wash. When done, moisturize your body with a fragrant lotion. Manicure your toes and hands.
- Sit by a cozy fireplace and cuddle with a good book or magazines with lots of beautiful pictures. Play enjoyable music in the background.
- Go to afternoon tea with a friend.
- Enjoy stained-glass windows in a church or chapel when the light is shining through them.
- Watch the sunset at the ocean and walk barefoot along the shoreline.
- Push a cart up and down the aisles of a supermarket or drug store, distracting your mind with the variety of different things on the shelves.

7. Invest in Yourself

One of the symptoms of depression is a lack of interest in the things you used to enjoy. This means you are going to have to be intentional to keep up with the meaningful activities in your life, such as getting together with friends, enjoying hobbies, going places, and having fun. This will take some effort, but staying isolated and inactive will only hinder and complicate your recovery. And remember, caring for and nurturing yourself is a vital component to your healing. Don't feel guilty if you pamper yourself or take time for rest and restoration.

Here are some ideas that have worked for other women: do something nice for yourself; take a long hot bath; buy yourself flowers; enjoy a place of beauty; take some extended time for something meaningful spiritually; talk with a friend; watch a funny movie; get some fresh air and sunlight; take a walk; listen to uplifting praise music; wear clothes that make you feel good; put on perfume, makeup, jewelry, and do your hair. Do anything that would be positive and enjoyable

8. Invest in Others

Do an act of kindness for someone else. Be available to listen or help out. My dear friend Beth, who is recovering from severe cancer, told me about how one evening she received a meal of homemade enchiladas for dinner. She was taken aback, because the woman who had made them was going through a very difficult time herself. She told Beth that she was having a bad day and decided to do something kind for someone else who was having a hard time as well. This helped her to feel better.

Many studies have reported that altruism (doing something kind for others) has benefits in depression recovery. When you care for yourself as well as someone else who may need your support, it helps you keep some perspective on the suffering of others and get your mind off your own problems. Doing something kind for someone else who is having a hard time will also make you feel better about yourself, because when you give, you also receive a blessing in return.

Overcoming the Roadblocks to Recovery

If only the road to recovery from depression was smooth sailing. Unfortunately, it isn't. There are many pitfalls, roadblocks, and challenges. Next, we will describe some of these challenges and offer help in negotiating them.

1. Be Prepared for Possible Setbacks

Don't expect too much from yourself and try not to be disappointed or give up when you have a setback. You are

Depression Survival Kit

Just for fun, pack yourself the following depression "survival kit." Put all these goodies in a clear bag, to help you remember that God can help you keep it all together!

A **candle** to remind you that even when you are surrounded by darkness, Christ's love is a fire that never goes out!

A **match** to remind you that sleep, relaxation, and exercise "re-light your flame" when you feel burned out!

A **band aid** to remind you that God comforts and heals, and that recovery takes time!

Two paper clips joined together to remind you that connecting with God, yourself, family, friends, your community, and your Christian faith mean more than anything else.

A **pencil** to remind you to list your blessings, use a prayer journal daily, and "pencil in" time for what really matters.

An **eraser** to remind you to keep your life clean by being honest with yourself and others, asking for forgiveness, and forgiving others.

A **piece of fleece blanket** to remind you to nurture and take good care of yourself.

A **Hershey's Hugs** to remind you that you are loved! (Sorry, not to comfort yourself with chocolate!)

Chewing gum to remind you to stick with it, to persevere and keep going.

A **Snickers** to remind you that laughter is good medicine! (Okay, go ahead and have a piece of chocolate!)

not a failure. Setbacks are part of the process. Sometimes we will take a few steps forward and one step back. But stay committed to moving forward, growing, learning new skills, and choosing habits of a wellness lifestyle. Don't give up! When faced with negative emotions like exhaustion, worthlessness, helplessness, or hopelessness, remember that these are symptoms of depression. When your treatment starts becoming effective, these symptoms will eventually fade away.

Know what triggers depression for you and what the warning signs are. They might appear during times of chronic strain and stress. You may become distressed, your eating and sleeping habits may change, you may start feeling overwhelmed and emotionally irritable, and your relationships may become disconnected and conflicted. These are all warning signs for depression and should be immediately heeded.

When you see these depression warning signs, be ready. Know what stress relievers work for you, or work on feeling the emotions, expressing them constructively, or connecting in meaningful relationships so you can rely on these effective resources for recovering from depression again.

2. Be Open to Professional Treatment

Among some there is a stigma attached to seeing a psychiatrist or a psychologist, but this stigma is not justified. It only breeds resistance.

Remember, your inability to just snap out of it says a lot about the power of depression and nothing about your willpower or strength of character. Like pain, it is a signal to alert you that something is amiss. There is a strong physiological component to all depression that causes the chemical messengers in your brain to be off balance. These neurotransmitters will not be realigned by your own willpower or a quick "pick-me-upper" fix. It will require an intentional strategy of understanding what is needed to combat the depression, through the many resources that God has provided for healing. These could include the encouragement and guidance of another through Christian counseling, as well as the gift of antidepressant medication.

3. You Won't Snap out of Depression Right Away

Building resistance and resilience takes time. Recovery from depression will take time (maybe weeks or months), depending on the root causes and effective treatment, along with your wellness lifestyle choices. Some symptoms may go away rather quickly, but others may not. To put it into perspective, it takes some time after having a baby for the body to readjust. In addition, if you suffer some significant loss, your grieving will take time. And when it comes to antidepressants, it may be a few weeks to a month before you notice any changes at all. Don't get frustrated if you aren't seeing immediate improvement. Realize you will need to persevere in doing what's helpful, and eventually the depression will lift.

4. Let Depression Go Once It Has Passed

For a small percentage of depression sufferers, the depression becomes "dividend paying." In other words, they get so used to being depressed that they don't give it up when the depression has actually lifted. They may continue to believe and behave as if they are depressed, because the depression pays them a "dividend" or bonus. In some cases, the dividend of depression means that family members, even a husband, treats them with kindness, or that they get their way by manipulating life around being depressed or incapacitated.

Depression can be maladaptive manipulation, giving a sense of power over situations and people. It can be used to punish those around us or to force them to have to change. So, truly desiring healing and recovery might require an honest look at what purpose it has served you, and how you can courageously let go of this misconception to keep moving toward experiencing healing and freedom.

5. Your Medication Could "Poop Out"

If you are on antidepressants, be sure to alert your doctor of any changes in your progress, as your body can adjust to the medication. Switching to something else will be necessary. See chapter 8 for more details.

6. The Symptoms of Depression Can Make It Difficult for You to Be Intentional and Proactive

Since depression can leave you with feelings of hopelessness and helplessness, low physical energy, lack of interest in life, isolation, negative thoughts, and sadness, the symptoms alone can be a serious challenge to taking care of yourself and getting the help you need. But be kind to yourself. Move forward without berating yourself for the symptoms of depression you are experiencing.

It's important to know the difference between taking some time out, which might be necessary especially around issues of loss, and just giving in to the symptoms and letting them rule your life. This is where the meaningful, trusting relationships in your life can be helpful. Family, friends, and a counselor can help you stay motivated, as well as help you discern when you need to take action and when you just need a break.

You Can Do It

Despite these obstacles, it is possible to achieve a full recovery and, more importantly, to build resistance to future depression. There is a high risk for repeated episodes of depression in those who are vulnerable. Successfully treating a current episode is winning half the battle. The total victory includes preventing future episodes as well.

However, throughout this book we have presented you with resources to get the help you need as soon as possible and to continue building resilience and resistance to prevent future episodes. Remember: The most effective strategy for recovery is an integrative approach—treating you as a whole person. Utilize medical resources, counseling, social support, natural therapies, and a wellness lifestyle. Take good care of yourself now.

May God bless you.

11

Caring for a Woman Who Is Depressed

Lord Jesus Christ, and God my father, who loves me and gives me everlasting consolation and encouragement, please encourage me and strengthen me in everything I say and do.

Prayer inspired by 2 Thessalonians 2:16–17

This chapter is intended primarily for husbands, but much of the information provided here could be useful for anyone trying to help a depressed mother, grandmother, daughter, or friend. The only difference is the intensity of your emotional involvement as you approach the problem.

As you work through this material, then, remember that any references to "husband" or "wife" are only a general guideline.

Nobody Suffers Alone

At the outset, let's agree that being around a depressed person, whether male or female, isn't easy. However, the quality of the relationship you develop can make all the difference in the world. A solid relationship will persevere, and even after the depression is over, will remain intact and strong. As a rule, however, the more serious the depression, the greater the potential strain on that relationship. Make no mistake about it; the struggle within every person who has a depressed loved one is agonizing. You long for your wife, mother, daughter, or friend to be back to normal again. You're afraid to put any more demands on her, yet you can't help but be angry at the state she's in. But remember this: You're not alone. You join with many, many others who have had to bear a similar burden.

The thing is, being around a depressed woman doesn't just take an emotional toll; it can take a physical one, as well. It's not uncommon for the caregiver of a depressed loved one to succumb to some illness himself, even to a serious depression, following a protracted period of caregiving. Intense caregiving is itself the source of great stress, and stress is bad for everything, including our immune systems.

That aside, the very nature of depression—especially its seeming resistance to any advice or counsel—easily creates a state of frustration and alienation in those who love the depressed person the most. It isn't necessarily a personal threat or offense. You see how she hurts herself, and you can't help getting angry. It's difficult to control your temper when a close relative or friend becomes self-neglectful or never returns your calls, only answers you in monosyllables, acts completely self-absorbed, or seems to have no appreciation for anything you do to help.

Research has shown that those who are around a depressed woman with a negative attitude experience significantly more conflict. It makes sense, since there is likely to be increased arguing and less direct communication. Family and friends around depressed women also feel frustrated, sad, and angry, not only with the depressed person, but also with themselves. Those who are closest to them also tend to feel angry, discouraged, and strained by the depressed person's fatigue, lack of interest in others, hopelessness, and irritability. No wonder these family and friends also have a much higher rate of anxiety and depressed moods themselves.[1]

The Dark before the Dawn

This might be the first episode of depression you've lived with. If it is, you will soon discover just how your frustration level can grow with time. And the more you try to be supportive and help her overcome her depression, the worse it seems to get.

This is an interesting phenomenon about serious depression: It always worsens before it gets better. A good analogy is how the night is darkest just before the dawn. In other words, some of the deepest depression will be seen during the weeks before the antidepressant takes effect. The person on the antidepressant becomes slightly hopeful that the medication will help, but as the weeks pass and nothing improves, she feels a greater sense of loss, and this often deepens the depression. This is one of the reasons why there is an increased risk of suicide while waiting for medication to kick in. Often, the medication is blamed for this increase. However, it's not the medication that is increasing the despair, but rather the expectations of the sufferer and those around her.

So, while waiting for the medication to take effect, do your best to remain optimistic, but keep it realistic. Healing will take time, so don't increase your frustration, or the frustration of your depressed loved one, by becoming impatient.

It's natural to feel that there is not much you can do that is helpful. It's common to wish that she would just "get over it." You have probably tried giving good advice, suggesting ways of "fixing it" and problem solving. You may also have cried with her and gone the extra mile many times over, but nothing has worked. And then there are those well-meaning people who have glibly told you, "Don't take it personally." They just don't realize how difficult it can be living with someone who is depressed. "Not taking it personally" is easier said than done. Frankly, you can't help but take it personally, and the more you love your depressed partner, the more personal it's going to feel. It's very difficult controlling your temper, frustration, sadness, and loneliness when the one you love so much seems to be hurting herself and inadvertently hurting those around her, as well.

Depressed women can also evoke a lot of guilt in those close to them. Loved ones begin to think, "Nothing I do seems to help, so there must be something wrong with me." But there's nothing wrong with the one trying to help, so there's no point in feeling guilty. This is, in all respects, a false guilt. There is nothing you can do to remove another's depression. No amount of love and understanding will, of themselves, make depression go away. However, love and patience are important, and there's a lot you can do to love and nurture her by attending to little things for her. Don't try to "fix" her yourself, but leave the treatment to the professionals. Concentrate on being available, empathetic, and responsive, making your reactions to your loved one's depression as healthy as you can. And don't forget to take good care of yourself.

Strategies for Helping a Depressed Loved One or Friend

There are several ways you can help a depressed loved one, and they don't have to be complex or difficult to implement. The simplest act of kindness can make a dif-

ference, even if it seems that the depressed loved one neither notices nor cares.

1. Develop a Strategy for Listening and Communicating

What is the most important thing you can do for a
depressed wife, mother, daughter, or friend? Without a
doubt, it is to listen and communicate love and acceptance
with all the power you can muster. Remember that your
feelings don't matter nearly as much as your behavior. You
may not feel the least bit loving, and this is understand-
able given your circumstances. But you can behave in a
loving manner. Read 1 Corinthians 13, that great chapter
on love. If you behave in a loving way, sooner or later your
feelings will return. For now, concentrate on doing loving
things. Be patient and understanding. Avoid blaming her
or being judgmental about her depression.

Start by frequently asking her how she's doing. Depressed people want to talk about how bad they feel, so
let her. And when she starts to talk, don't cut her off.
What she may need more than anything is just to talk,
cry, and have you listen and say, "I'm so sorry you are so
sad today, but the time will come when you will be happy
again." Just hold her and let her cry on your shoulder.
Don't feel like you have to fix her or make things better.
Just be there. Say "I love you, and I'm sorry you're sad.
Keep talking and telling me what's wrong and how you
are feeling."

A depressed woman needs a listening ear, understanding, patience, acceptance, and love. Granted, this can be
very difficult to provide, because when women are
depressed, they can be very frustrating and uncomfortable to be around. Men, in contrast, like to fix tribulations
and give advice. Their instinctive response is to solve problems. But a problem-solving attitude, unless you are the

professional treating her, is not what she wants or needs. That will only create more frustration and add to the woman's negative feelings of inadequacy, despair, and hopelessness.

Remind yourself often that your loved one has not chosen to be depressed. Disappointing as this truth may be, try to accept her depression and its impact on your life with patience and grace. Remember that depression saps energy and diminishes self-esteem, and it will make your loved one feel worthless and unwanted. Guilt hangs heavy and low over every depressed woman's life, and thoughts of dying are very common. Unconditional love can make all the difference in the long run to both you and your depressed loved one. Even though she may never show any appreciation for it while she is depressed, the day will come when you will look back with great satisfaction over how you handled your reactions.

Until then, make time to listen, talk, and share feelings. Depressed people tend to withdraw and isolate themselves. It's part of what depression does to you. Your wife may not be the one to initiate talking, much less anything else. Therefore, you must be prepared to take the initiative. You can never go wrong by just asking her how she is feeling. She may not talk readily about what is bothering her, but by simply allowing her to speak what's on her mind, she may eventually come to express and understand her own feelings.

We realize that this is going to be very difficult for some of you (especially men who like to solve and fix problems). Empathy, however, means taking her perspective into consideration. Walking in her shoes "for a mile or two," as Will Rogers used to say, will change your perspective and build love between the two of you.

What we are emphasizing here is the importance of really trying to understand how your loved one has to struggle to get through each day. Ask her about these struggles, so that you can be as empathic as possible. Ask yourself whether you have ever felt similarly. If you haven't, then try to imagine feeling that way now. Tell her how painful it feels for you to simply imagine being in her condition yourself.

Since it is quite common for men not to understand what empathy is all about, here are some examples of what an empathic response should be:

- You must really feel spent after such a hard day with the kids.
- I know it must really hurt you when your mom says those things to you.
- It sounds like you are feeling really angry.

Try to reflect back what she is saying. Often, what people say or how they act doesn't communicate what they are really meaning or feeling. "Reflective listening," the sort of listening that constantly "checks out" the accuracy of what one is hearing, is a powerful empathy-building tool. So, say what it is you think you heard your loved one say. If she corrects you, try again with the new bit of information. Try to convey that you really understand her feelings, especially the feelings beneath the surface reactions. Don't try to suggest ways she can get over her bad feelings. This comes across as a judgment, even a rejection. It's more important to acknowledge what you have heard and be more sensitive to her feelings and needs.

And speaking of being sensitive, here are a few things you should never say to the depressed woman in your life:

- Its all your own fault you're depressed. Pull yourself together.

- There must be something wrong with your spiritual life. God must not be pleased with you at the moment. Maybe you have unforgiven sins.
- Stop feeling so sorry for yourself and just try a little harder. You're just being lazy.
- I don't know how much more of this I can take. You're driving me crazy.
- Remember that there are many people in this world who are worse off than you.
- I'm beginning to think that it was a mistake for me to marry you.
- You should stop seeing those quacks and taking those pills because they're just a cop out and are changing your brain.
- Believe me, I know how you feel because I was depressed once, but I didn't make such a big deal of it. Just snap out of it.
- You have everything going for you. You have nothing to be sad about. You should be having the time of your life. You don't 'look' depressed.
- It will be okay. I know, I understand.
- Snap out of it. Get out and get some fresh air. Take some time to reevaluate.

So what should you say? Try a few of these:

- I love you and always will because you are important to me.
- I admit that I don't understand the pain or feelings you are experiencing, but I will love you and support you through this time.
- You don't have to apologize for the way you feel, because I know that it's due to the depression.

- You are not alone in this, I will stand with you until it's over. I will not abandon you.
- Do you want a hug? I love you.
- I'll do whatever it takes to help you. I am going to be a support to you.
- Let me hold you and listen to you while you share your feelings and cry.
- Some of God's greatest servants have also suffered from depression. God didn't cause it and he helped them through; he'll help you through as well.
- If you're not up to it, let me make the phone call to the doctor and make sure you get to your appointment.

2. Learn Everything You Can about Depression Yourself

The second major strategy for helping someone who is depressed is to learn all you can about depression. This may seem a strange assignment, but there are several reasons for it. First, the more you understand about what causes depression, the less likely you will be to make it worse. Ignorance about the causes of depression only serves to aggravate it. You will say and do the wrong things. You will blame your spouse for something she is not responsible for. Second, the more you understand what depression does, the more patient and kind you will become. The third reason is that the more you know about depression, the less helpless you will feel about not being able to control it. In fact, this has an empowering effect on the loved ones of those who are depressed. Last, the more you know, the more hopeful you will feel. Depression is no longer the mystifying, uncontrollable beast it used to be, so plunging into research on the subject and learning everything you can may be the most positive way to cope. The "unknown" can be very stressful.

3. Be Supportive in Practical Ways

To be supportive to a loved one as she tries to overcome her depression means creating a safe, nurturing environment — and to do this in practical ways as well. Recovering from depression takes time. The antidepressants take at least two weeks to take effect after the dosage is high enough, and may take several months for the full effect to be seen. In some cases, it may be necessary to try out several combinations of medication before the right mix is found. It's possible that six months could pass before the depression lifts. And it's during this waiting period that a depressed woman needs all the love, patience, encouragement, and practical support that can be mobilized.

Daily chores can be particularly threatening. Remember that the symptoms of depression include pessimism, lethargy, and anhedonia, or the inability to derive any pleasure or enjoyment out of life. These symptoms, then, can make otherwise simple tasks seem insurmountable. You can help not just by being positive and hopeful, but also by relieving your loved one of those practical tasks that she can't handle right now. You must be both available and accessible in very practical ways, including helping with housework, washing, cooking a meal (or going out for dinner occasionally), or offering to take care of the kids while your wife gets a manicure, goes to the salon, or some other personal treat. And if you can't personally help out with these chores because of business or work demands, then ask a relative or friend, or employ someone to "stand in" for you. Not only are these symbols of your love, but they are also helpful, practical ways you can bring relief to your wife. For the time being, she can't fulfill even her own expectations, let alone yours.

Practical Ways You Can Help a Depressed Loved One

1. Listen to and talk with her about how she feels and experiences her depression.
2. If she is reluctant to talk to you, which is possible, encourage her to talk to a reliable, trustworthy friend.
3. If you have children, offer to take the children one evening or weekend so she can have a night off with a friend. Offer to take the kids for a day, so she can have a day alone at home to take care of personal needs.
4. Offer to make the evening meal often, or to take care of household chores around the house. Remember: She is not just being lazy. Depression robs you of all energy.
5. Suggest making appointments for her, and offer to take her to these so she doesn't have to go alone.
6. Offer to arrange for child care to give her a break from regular duties or to take care of personal needs. (Don't take complete ownership of your loved one's condition yourself. She must have some investment in getting well, or she will resist the process. It is important not to rescue her, but be available to help out.)
7. Remind and encourage her to keep doctors' appointments, continue with medication, and pursue wellness living. (Depression upsets memory, so it can be easy to forget these.)
8. Keep reaching out to her. Show that you care by calling her on the phone; inviting her out to the movies, ball games, parties, or church; send her little notes of love. Don't be discouraged if she does not respond to your gestures. Your efforts will be noticed and eventually, as she recovers, she will respond.
9 Pray with her and for her. There is no greater source of comfort than prayer.

4. Don't Leave Her to Fight Her Depression on Her Own

Depression is about the loneliest experience anyone can have. No one can enter that world with you; you're on your own, or so it seems. But you can be there for a depressed one and keep her connected to healing and recovery resources, as well as whatever social support you can muster. In particular, it is very important for her to have female friends or family members that she can confide in on a daily basis. Continuous support and encouragement will, at the least, remind her that she's not alone. Research is very clear on this point: Social support helps to improve treatment results and speed up recovery.

Depression is a "whole person" illness. Unlike, say, a broken leg that may affect your mobility, depression affects every part of your being, including the emotional, physical, and spiritual. Recovery, therefore, requires an integrative approach. Treatment focuses not just on recovery, but also on building resistance and resilience to overcome future depression.

Role Changes and Considerations

We have listed some of the practical ways you can support your depressed loved one. But there are also other changes, including role changes, that can challenge relationships, especially between husband and wife.

Depression alters the roles each plays in a marriage, and this can affect your family life as well. You may have to take over responsibilities normally undertaken by your wife, mother, or daughter, such as: doing the grocery shopping; paying the bills; driving the kids to and from school and afternoon activities; preparing evening meals; feeding the animals; cleaning up after the animals; and coordinating daily household chores like cleaning floors, washing the dishes, and doing the laundry. These are all unavoidable role changes that have to be made.

In particular, you will need to think about how you will deal with your children. Children easily take responsibility for their parent's unhappiness. They can even be made to feel guilty for the pain they see, becoming more vulnerable to depression themselves. Reassure the children that they are not responsible for their mother's depression, that it is not their fault, and that they can't fix it. Reassure them that although their mom is not well right now, she is getting help and will soon be back to normal. It is particularly important to educate them about how depression can be a biological condition that needs treatment, just as an illness like diabetes needs to be treated. Unfortunately, there is a strong bias in our culture, born of ignorance, that stigmatizes an emotional problem like depression just because we can't "see" the cause of the problem. A father should make it perfectly clear that their mother is not suffering from anything strange or weird, but from an illness as real as any other.

If necessary, make supplementary arrangements to ensure that your children's basic needs are being met. Cover all the bases to make sure nothing falls through the cracks. This might include having a friend or grandparent prepare lunches for their school, help with homework, or get them to and from school, sporting activities, and health care. Try to maintain a life as normal as possible for the children, without making your wife feel that she is failing in her duties.

There is one very important consideration we would like to mention here, as it is often overlooked, not just by parents, but by professionals as well: Children and teenagers can be at risk for increased depression themselves when someone as close as their mother is seriously depressed.

How can you recognize the symptoms of depression in children? While some children show it in the conventional way of sadness and crying, often it is masked by increased acting out and disruptive behavior. To put it succinctly, depressed children can become angry at both seeing their mother in pain and the loss of their mother's warmth and closeness. Watch for the following typical symptoms of depression in children and teenagers:

- Persistent sadness
- Loss of interest or pleasure in activities that once were enjoyable
- Decreased appetite
- Inability to fall asleep or early wakening
- Frequent physical complaints such as headaches, stomachaches, or tiredness
- Talk of or attempts to run away from home
- Outbursts of shouting or crying, irritability, anger, or displays of hostility

Some of the more atypical symptoms of depression in children and teenagers include:

- Feeling bitter in response to positive events
- Increased appetite and overeating
- Weight gain
- Excessive sleepiness or sleeping
- Slower motor movement or reactions
- Difficulty in relationships and making conversation, and social isolation

What should you do if you suspect that your child is also becoming depressed? If the depression appears serious to the extent that your child won't go to school or just lies around moping, we recommend you seek professional help right away. If the child's reactions seem minor, then reassurance and some additional attention from you and the rest of your extended family could help allay your child's fears.

Social Adjustments

There are other changes that will also have to be made during the period of a wife's depression. A couple's social life will certainly need adjusting. This does not mean disconnecting from normal social activities or becoming isolated, but rather being selective about what social activities you engage in. Above all else, a husband should try to avoid situations that could be embarrassing to his wife. No wife who is depressed wants her depression to be on display. When your social skills are temporarily disabled, you don't want to be humiliated in front of others.

A visit to the movies may have to replace the opera, or going to church may mean sitting at the back and slipping out before anyone else. You may have to temporarily surrender certain couple friendships that are straining, or decline dinner invitations that will be too uncomfortable. Social demands can create excessive additional stress that can aggravate the depression of your loved one. When not able to attend social events, you don't have to apologize. You can simply explain that she is experiencing a period of depression and that during her recovery time, out of consideration for her well-being, you are limiting your social schedule so as not to add stress.

Try to find new rituals, routines, and ways of connecting with others. A word of caution here, however. While your wife may be unresponsive during her depression, avoid the temptation to share your feelings intimately with another woman. The lure to seek out a sympathetic ear may be quite strong when intimacy is limited. This is dangerous territory and can make you vulnerable to an affair. Rather, choose to share your feelings with a family member, male friend, your pastor, or a professional therapist. One of the sacrifices that a loving husband must be willing to make when his wife is depressed is to forego sexual intimacy, if needed. The real test of a man's character, and faith, might well be in this area. God understands what a sacrifice this may mean and will honor it.

Take Good Care of Yourself

Don't underestimate the importance of daily lifestyle basics of eating well, getting enough sleep, exercising, relaxing, and staying connected with God and others. These mundane daily choices are essential strategies that will give you the energy and basic resources as a whole person to deal with the strain and stress of helping your loved one through this difficult time. Any one of these basics of life being off balance could deplete you of necessary patience, clarity of mind, hope, energy, or restoration that allow you to be a help to your partner and keep you from being negatively impacted by the depression. It may help your partner if you initiate, for example, proper sleeping patterns, relaxation, and healthy eating, and commit to these together.

Find a New Routine and Keep with It As Much As Possible

Another way to maintain your ability to be helpful and guard against your vulnerability to depression is to keep up with your hobbies, interests, and work, and stay connected to the meaningful people in your life. Have fun.

These can all help manage your stress and minimize your anger and resentment for the depression affecting your life. You will also then be able to be more helpful and supportive of your loved one.

Stay Connected with Social Support

Stay involved with other people. Avoid being isolated, spending most of your time alone or only with the depressed loved one. Solidify and rely on meaningful relationships with family and friends. Keep up with regular golfing with the "buddies," meeting for breakfast once a week in the morning with a friend, "doing lunch," going to card night, attending prayer meetings, and keeping up with other meaningful social interactions. Being around other nondepressed, positive people will recharge you, keep you protected from the weariness of depression symptoms, and guard you against depression yourself. Ask others to pray for her and you, as she overcomes and recovers from depression.

Several research studies have shown that when caregivers struggle on their own, isolated from anyone else who can understand and support them, they burn out quickly on an emotional level. A social support system also provides a better perspective on what you're suffering, and this helps you to be a better caregiver. Lastly, a social support system provides a safe place for you to express your feelings and experience comfort and encouragement.

Ask for Help

Besides the individual friendships you already have, how about building a support group? You have several choices. Ask a few friends if they would be willing to meet with you, say, over breakfast for an hour a week. Offer to be a support to them at the same time they will be supporting you. There isn't a person on this planet who isn't struggling with some personal challenge at some point in time. You can approach a counselor or psychotherapist in your area and see if he or she has any groups that could serve as a support. Lastly, you can see a therapist for individual "support," if only on a biweekly or monthly basis. This has the advantage of having someone who can support you and monitor your own risk for depression and potential for burnout.

Retain Intimacy

It is important, as well, that you maintain a sense of connection in your relationship, even if you feel that you are being pushed away. Even if your intimate giving isn't reciprocated, give it nevertheless. Hold her hands whenever you can. Touch her cheek and tell her you love her. Hold her close so that she can feel your warmth.

A couple often needs help from a professional therapist with this, as it is difficult to find the meaning of actions, understand the core emotions, and have an objective viewpoint of the other person.

Just for the One Who Is Depressed

Our closing comments are directed at the reader who is depressed. It's not easy to live with depression. It's not easy to live in this world when you are depressed. It's not easy to be loving, decent, and kind when you walk every day with such deep emotional pain. It's not easy to understand yourself, to just be yourself, or even to like yourself. But you have to go on living no matter what it feels like. You have to live with yourself and those you love, and the only way you can do this with dignity is to ensure that you are doing everything in your power to bring healing as soon as you can.

So make peace with yourself, your guilt, and your need to please everybody else. You are accountable to no one except God himself, and he understands perfectly what you are going through.

For this brief period of time, focus only on your own healing. With God's help, this period of sadness and despair could turn out to be a time of glorious partnership with God's eternal purposes. It is in these moments of deep hurt that God does his finest work in us—if we are willing to surrender.

Notes

Chapter 1

1. Daniel Goleman, "A Rising Cost of Modernity: Depression," *New York Times*, Dec. 8, 1992; "The Changing Rate of Major Depression," *Journal of the American Medical Association* 268, no. 21 (1992): 3098–3105.

2. Martin E.P. Seligman. *What You Can Change . . . And What You Can't* (New York: Fawcett Columbine, 1995), 105-107.

3. Richard A. Swenson, M.D. *Margin: Restoring Emotional, Physical, Financial, and Time Reserves to Overloaded Lives.* (Colorado Springs: NavPress, 1993), 102

4. S. Gilied, and S. Kofman. "Women and Mental Health" (Issues for health reform background paper.) New York: The Commonwealth Fund, Commission on Women's Health.

Chapter 2

1. www.wingofmadness.com

2. "Depression May Hinder Health Care," *Prevention,* August, 2000.

Chapter 3

1. *Archives of General Psychiatry* 42 (1985): 689

2. "Hidden Cause of Fatigue, Nervousness and Depression," *Prevention,* August, 2000.

3. Brenda Poinsett. *Why Do I Feel This Way?* (Colorado Springs: NavPress, 1996), 58.

Chapter 4

1. Judith Viorst. *Necessary Losses* (New York: Tawcett, 1986), 22.

2. Richard O. O'Connor, Ph.D. *Undoing Depression* (New York: Berkley, 1997), 107.

Chapter 5

1. Richard A. Swenson, M.D. *Margin: Restoring Emotional, Physical, Financial, and Time Reserves to Overloaded Lives* (Colorado Springs: NavPress, 1992), 61.

2. www.healthywomen.org, November 2000 posting

3. Shelley Taylor, Ph.D., along with five colleagues at the University of California, Los Angeles.

Chapter 6

1. "The National Longitudinal Study on Adolescent Health," *Journal of the American Medical Association* in (1997).
2. Arlene Eisenberg. *What to Expect When You're Expecting* (New York: Workman, 1996), 398–400.

Chapter 7

1. www.amft.org Consumer Update: Depression Volume1 Issue 2 March 1999.
2. Dr. Archibald D. Hart and Dr. Timothy Hogan. *How to Find the Help You Need* (Grand Rapids: Zondervan, 1996), 61.
3. G. L. Klerman and M. M. Wiseman. "Interpersonal Therapy," *E. S. Paykel Hanbook of Affective Disorders* (New York: Guilford, 1992), 96.

Chapter 9

1. In her book *EVEolution: The Eight Truths of Marketing to Women,* Faith Popcorn states that women have created a $9.8 billion pharmacopoeia for alternative medicine.
2. Varro E. Tyler, Ph.D. "St. John's Wort Update," *Prevention,* August, 2000.
3. Jean Carper. *Your Miracle Brain* (New York: HarperCollins, 2000), 295-298.
4. Richard Brown, M.D., Teodoro Bottiglieri, Ph.D., and Carol Colman. *Stop Depression Now* (New York: Berkley, 2000).
5. Syd Baumel. *Dealing with Depression Naturally* (Los Angeles: Keats Publishing, 2000), 115–118.
6. Michael T. Murray. *Natural Alternatives to Prozac* (New York: William Marrow and Company Inc., 1996), 174.
7. Sara M. Rosenthal. *Women and Depression* (Los Angeles: Lowell House, 2000), 186.
8. *American Journal of Psychiatry,* vol 154 (1997).
9. Michael Murray, M.D. and Joseph Pizzaro, M.D. *Encyclopedia of Natural Medicine* (Rocklin, Ca.: Prima Health Publishing, 1998).
10. www.advancedbrain.com

Chapter 11

1. Laura Epstein Rosen, Ph.D., and Xavier Francisco Amador, Ph.D. *When Someone You Love Is Depressed* (New York: Simon and Schuster, 1997), 5 –6.

Resources

There are many great books available that will be helpful to you, but here are a few to begin with. Please use discretion. Not all books listed here are from an exclusively Christian perspective, however helpful information can still be gleaned. Books with an * are not primarily Christian.

Books

Depression

Baumel, Syd. *Dealing with Depression Naturally.* Los Angeles: Keats, 2000.*

Cousens, Gabriel, M.D. *Depression Free for Life.* New York: HarperCollins, 2000.*

Moore, Beth. *Praying God's Word.* Nashville: Broadman & Holman, 2000.

Moore, Pam Rosewell. *When Spring Comes Late: Finding Your Way through Depression.* Grand Rapids: Chosen Books, 2000.

O'Conner, Richard, Ph.D. *Undoing Depression.* New York: Little, Brown and Company, 1997.*

Poinsett, Brenda. *Why Do I Feel This Way?* Colorado Springs: NavPress, 1996.

Raskin, Valerie Davis, M.D. *When Words Are Not Enough: The Woman's Prescription for Depression and Anxiety.* New York: Broadway, 1997.*

Rosen, Laura Epstein, Ph.D. and Xavier Francisco Amador, Ph.D. *When Someone You Love Is Depressed: How to Help Your Loved One without Loosing Yourself.* New York: Fireside, 1997.*

Rosenthal, M. Sara. *Women & Depression.* Los Angeles: Lowell House, 2000.*

Stress and Anxiety

Bloomfield, Harold H., M.D. *Healing Anxiety Naturally.* New York: HarperCollins, 1998.*

Hart, Archibald, Ph.D. *Adrenaline and Stress.* Dallas: Word, 1995.

———. *The Anxiety Cure.* Dallas: Word, 1999.

Seligman, Martin E. P., Ph.D. *What You Can Change—and What You Can't.* New York: Fawcett, 1993.*

Swenson, Richard A., M.D. *Margin.* Colorado Springs: NavPress, 1992.

Physical

Hart, Archibald, Ph.D.; Debra Taylor, M.A.; and Catherine Weber, Ph.D. *Secrets of Eve: Understanding the Mystery of Female Sexuality.* Nashville: Word, 1998.

Mayo, Mary Ann and Joseph L. Mayo, M.D. *The Menopause Manager.* Grand Rapids: Revell, 1998.

Murray, Michael, N.D. and Joseph Pizzorno N.D. *Encyclopedia of Natural Medicine.* Rocklin, Calif.: Prima Health, 1998.*

Mind/Emotions

Burns, D. David, M.D. *The Feeling Good Handbook.* New York: Penguin Putnam, 1999.*

Seamands, David A. and Beth Funk. *Healing for Damaged Emotions Workbook.* Colorado Springs: Chariot Victor, 1992.

Websites

These are not all Christian websites, so please use discretion when getting information and advice from these websites.
Search for the topic of *depression* and *women,* or other related interests on these sites:

www.christian-depression.org
www.christianlifeskills.com
www.geocities.com/melministry
www.mentalhelp.net
www.nutritionalsupplements.com
www.webmd.com
www.psychcentral.com
www.undoingdepression.com
www.mayohealth.org
www.prevention.com
www.WholeHealthMD.com
www.drkoop.com
www.psycom.net/depression.central.women.html
www.pharmweb.net
www.nimh.nig.gov (National Institute of Mental Health)
www.mentalhealth.org
www.archibaldhart.com (Dr. Hart's website)
www.catherinehartweber.com (Dr. Weber's website)

Catherine Hart Weber, Ph.D.

Catherine received a Bachelors of Science from U.C.L.A., a Masters in Christian Leadership from Fuller Theological Seminary, and a Ph.D. in Marriage and Family Therapy from Fuller Graduate School of Psychology, Pasadena, California. She is a licensed marriage and family therapist, specializing in psychotherapy from a Christian perspective.

Catherine co-authored the *Secrets of Eve: Understanding the Mystery of Female Sexuality,* which reports the recent national study on Christian Female Sexuality which she participated in conducting.

Catherine researches, writes, speaks, and consults on topics relating to marriage enrichment, sexuality, the personal life of leaders, wellness for women, and integrative health.

Catherine is married to Rick, and has two daughters, Nicole and Caitlan, who keep her life very full. They live in the foothill village of Sierra Madre, California, where Catherine enjoys getting fresh air and sunlight by walking in the hills with her golden retriever, Honey, and cultivating her English and vegetable gardens, as well as her friendships.

Archibald D. Hart, Ph.D.

Dr. Hart is currently Senior Professor of Psychology and Dean Emeritus of the Graduate School of Psychology,

Fuller Theological Seminary, Pasadena, California. He also serves as the executive editor and director of international relations for the American Association of Christian Counselors, a forty thousand member organization with members from all around the world.

Originally trained in South Africa, he joined the faculty at the Graduate School of Psychology, Fuller Theological Seminary, in May 1973. He is licensed in the state of California as a psychologist and board certified in Psychopharmacology. He specializes in psychotherapy from a Christian orientation, the treatment of depression, anxiety, and stress disorders. He was the first recipient in 1978 of the Weyerhaeuser Award for Faculty Excellence given by Fuller Theological Seminary.

Dr. Hart, often together with his wife Kathleen, lectures widely to church groups and ministers on topics of the personal life of the minister, marriage, stress in children, stress management, emotions and how to handle them from a Christian point of view, the affects of divorce on children, and the emotional hazards of ministry, focusing on the personal life of the pastor and spouse.

He enjoys a broad range of creative activities from jewelry making and electronic inventions to cooking recipes from his international travels. He and Kathleen have three daughters and seven grandchildren whom they enjoy thoroughly.